Examination of the Newborn

Newborn babies are examined at around 6 to 72 hours after their birth to rule out major congenital abnormalities and reassure the parents that their baby is healthy. This practical text is a step-by-step guide for all practitioners who undertake this clinical examination. It is particularly valuable for midwives and nurses undertaking Examination of the Newborn modules as well as a useful reference work for those already performing this role. It provides midwives and other practitioners involved in neonatal examination with a comprehensive guide to the holistic examination of the newborn infant.

Examination of the Newborn encourages the reader to view each mother and baby as unique, taking into account their experiences preconceptually, antenatally and through childbirth. The text covers:

- the role of the first examination as a screening tool;
- normal fetal development;
- parents' concerns and how to respond to them;
- the impact of antenatal diagnostic screening;
- the events of labour and birth;
- the clinical examination of the neonate;
- the identification and management of congenital abnormalities;
- accountability and legal issues.

This new edition is thoroughly revised throughout to meet current Nursing and Midwifery Council (NMC) and National Screening Committee standards. It includes a new chapter on the context and effectiveness of the examination and increased coverage of the impact of intrapartum management on the newborn, including fetal monitoring, place of birth, mode of birth and pain relief. Case scenarios, model answers, questions and further reading help the reader to apply the content to their own practice.

Helen Baston is Consultant Midwife: Public Health at Sheffield Teaching Hospitals NHS Trust, UK, a Supervisor of Midwives and Lecturer/Researcher at Sheffield Hallam University, UK.

Heather Durward is Associate Specialist in Paediatrics at Chesterfield Royal Hospital Foundation Trust, UK.

Examination of the Newborn

A practical guide

Second edition

Helen Baston and
Heather Durward

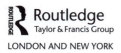
Routledge
Taylor & Francis Group

LONDON AND NEW YORK

First edition published 2001
by Routledge

This edition published 2010
by Routledge
2 Park Square, Milton Park, Abingdon, Oxon, OX14 4RN

Simultaneously published in the USA and Canada
by Routledge
270 Madison Avenue, New York, NY 10016

Routledge is an imprint of the Taylor & Francis Group, an informa business

© 2001, 2010 Helen Baston and Heather Durward

Typeset in Sabon by Prepress Projects Ltd, Perth, UK
Printed and bound in Great Britain by TJ International Ltd, Padstow, Cornwall

British Library Cataloguing in Publication Data
A catalogue record for this book is available from the British Library

Library of Congress Cataloging in Publication Data
Baston, Helen, 1962–
Examination of the newborn : a practical guide / Helen Baston and Heather
Durward. – 2nd ed.
p. ; cm.
Includes bibliographical references.
1. Newborn infants–Medical examinations. I. Durward, Heather, 1960– II.
Title.
[DNLM: 1. Physical Examination–methods. 2. Infant, Newborn. WS 141
B327e 2010]
RJ255.5.B37 2010
618.92'01–dc22
2009050218

ISBN10: 0-415-55162-5 (hbk)
ISBN10: 0-415-55163-3 (pbk)
ISBN10: 0-203-84995-7 (ebk)

ISBN13: 978-0-415-55162-5 (hbk)
ISBN13: 978-0-415-55163-2 (pbk)
ISBN13: 978-0-203-84995-8 (ebk)

For our husbands,
Simon and John,
and our beautiful children,
Hannah, Joseph and Sarah

Contents

Illustrations

Plates

Figures

Tables

Boxes

Preface to the second edition

This new text builds on the success of the first edition and now includes self-test exercises, activities and extra resources. It also includes a selection of colour plates to enhance the practitioner's identification of some major congenital abnormalities. *Examination of the Newborn: A Practical Guide* (second edition) brings together not only the clinical aspects of the examination but also the professional and legal frameworks that underpin this important screening event. It also encourages the practitioner to consider the woman and her family as unique, influenced by many factors, including social, economic and medical. This text does not replace the excellent sources of information found in individual chapters in larger texts but provides a valuable source of essential information within one compact volume. It will raise practitioners' awareness of the issues that relate to the first examination of the newborn and thus invoke a thirst for further reading of work referred to within the text.

Examination of the Newborn: A Practical Guide (second edition) offers all practitioners involved in undertaking this clinical role with a comprehensive framework with guidance for safe, effective care. The examination of the newborn has traditionally been undertaken by paediatric senior house officers or general practitioners and is now increasingly carried out by midwives and neonatal nurses. The roles of the midwife and neonatal nurse are expanding within neonatal care. Further educational opportunities have enabled practitioners to develop enhanced clinical skills in accordance with the frameworks defined by their regulatory body, which for nurses and midwives is the Nursing and Midwifery Council and for doctors is the General Medical Council. Such role expansion has become increasingly valuable as practitioners strive to enhance the quality of services that they provide. For example, since the publication of the document *Changing Childbirth* (Department of Health 1993a) midwives have explored ways that enable them to provide continuity of care to women and their families. One popular model is midwifery-led care, in which low-risk women are cared for by midwives who assume the role of lead professional. Medical support is requested only if a problem is identified. This system, however, often falls down in the postnatal period. Although fit and healthy postnatal women are often transferred into the community by midwives without medical input, this responsibility does not extend to the transfer of the baby. Thus, midwives are seeking to achieve competence to undertake the clinical examination of the neonate in order to provide a total package of care for low-risk women and their families.

The clinical examination of the newborn is also an issue because of the increasing number of home births, in line with the choice agenda advocated by government policy (Department of Health 2007). The majority of home births take place without medical cover, and general practitioners, who are not involved in intrapartum care, are sometimes unavailable or unable to perform this examination. Women are sometimes faced with a request to take their baby to the hospital to be examined, despite a normal pregnancy and labour (Thorpe-Raghdo 1995). Many midwives feel that they are ideally placed to undertake this role after undergoing appropriate education and supervised clinical practice.

This education is now a reality. Following the pioneering work of Stephanie Michaelides and colleagues at Middlesex University (Michaelides 1995), experienced neonatal nurses and midwives are able to access specific programmes that combine theory with clinical practice. Such educational provision also gives the practitioner the opportunity to look carefully at the role of the examination of the newborn infant and explore how it can be enhanced. It must be emphasised that the primary skill used by the practitioner when examining the neonate is the validation of normality. With increasing experience and knowledge, nursing and midwifery practitioners will be able to identify specific medical conditions; however, the *diagnosis* of abnormality remains the remit of the medical practitioner.

Examination of the Newborn: A Practical Guide (second edition) takes the examination of the newborn into a new phase, using a family-centred approach to this important consultation. This text encourages *all* practitioners with responsibility for the examination of the newborn to see each baby as unique, an individual born into a complex community. Although the chapters are related to each other, they are designed so that they can also be read independently.

Chapter 1 is a new addition and explores the evidence around effectiveness and competence of the neonatal examination. It discusses the evidence around who is best placed to undertake the examination and introduces the reader to national competencies.

Chapter 2 sets the scene for an individualised approach to the examination of the newborn baby. To do this the practitioner needs to consider preconceptual issues that affect women and how these may manifest during the examination of the baby. It alerts the examiner to the fact that each baby is the result of a unique combination of factors and that, through developing an appreciation of these, the examiner will be able to focus the examination to meet the specific needs of the family unit.

Chapter 3 considers normal fetal development in the light of the potential hazards to which the fetus may be exposed during its development. For the practitioner to be able to offer practical advice to women, an evidence-based approach to care is essential. This section provides a detailed look at the literature regarding the hazards to the fetus. It encourages the reader to develop strategies for answering the concerns voiced by parents during the examination.

Chapter 4 focuses on normal antenatal care and how fetal well-being is assessed. It highlights the dilemmas associated with antenatal diagnostic screening in order to provide the practitioner who examines the newborn with insight into the potential anxiety that may have been a dominant factor throughout the pregnancy.

Chapter 5 addresses some of the events that could occur during labour and birth and that could affect the health of the neonate. It also considers the implications of some of the choices that women make about how they would like their labour to be managed.

Chapter 6 takes the practitioner through the complete examination of the newborn, step by step, and focuses on the normal neonate.

Chapter 7 considers the most frequently encountered congenital abnormalities and describes their initial management.

Chapter 8 highlights the issues of accountability and medical negligence that are particularly important for the practitioner examining the newborn baby. It discusses the related aspects of care, such as informed consent and record keeping.

Examination of the Newborn: A Practical Guide (second edition) provides a comprehensive guide to the holistic examination of the newborn. It provides the practitioner with a resource of related literature and concludes with an appendix of national support groups.

Note to the reader

For convenience, the feminine third person pronoun will be used when referring to the practitioner, and the masculine third person pronoun when referring to the baby. This usage does not reflect any bias on the part of the authors.

Acknowledgements

We would like to express our gratitude to our families and friends whose support and encouragement have made this second edition possible. We continue to value the professional wisdom of colleagues who commented on the first edition of *Examination of the Newborn*, in particular Stephen Swan and Lesley Daniels. Ian Pickering remains a constant source of inspiration in striving for excellence in the provision of all aspects of health care. We would like to express our gratitude to Keith R. Walton for his sensitive artistic contribution to the illustrations in this text and to McGraw Hill for their permission to use the plates in this revised edition.

We would like to thank Khanam Virjee and Grace McInnes at Routledge for their encouragement, our copy-editor, Deborah Bennett, for her patient attention to detail, the production editor, Andrew R. Davidson, for his guidance, and our reviewers for their constructive comments.

Chapter 1   Examination of the newborn: where are we now?

- Introduction
- What is the examination of the newborn?
- Role of the examination as a screening tool
- Who should undertake the examination of the newborn?
- Examining effectiveness
- Education and competence
- Summary
- Self-test
- Activities
- Resources

Introduction

A comprehensive clinical examination is performed on all babies, usually within the first 72 hours of life. It consists of a full physical assessment to reassure parents that their baby is healthy, is fully developed and has no abnormalities. The examination is part of a range of post birth screening opportunities, which also include a midwife check immediately after birth; hearing testing; neonatal blood spot; and a further physical examination at 8 weeks of age. In this chapter we will consider the role of the examination as a screening tool, its effectiveness and the competence of practitioners.

What is the examination of the newborn?

This clinical examination comprises a top-to-toe physical examination of the baby and a clinical examination involving auscultation of the heart and lungs, detailed examination of the eye, palpation of the abdomen and assessment of the hips. It is performed in addition to the physical examination of the baby undertaken by midwives shortly after the birth of the baby. The National Institute for Health and Clinical Excellence (NICE) (2006) has stipulated the content of the examination (see Box 1.1). The person who undertakes the examination (the midwife, nurse or paediatrician) will be referred to as the *practitioner*. The examination itself goes by a range of titles, for example 'examination of the newborn' (Baston and Durward 2001; Townsend *et al*. 2004), the 'neonatal examination' (Hall 1999; Mitchell 2003), 'physical assessment of the newborn' (Lumsden 2002) or the 'newborn physical examination' [UK National Screening Committee (UK NCS) 2008a].

As the length of postnatal hospital stay has declined, this first examination is often combined with the traditional discharge examination that confirms the baby's fitness to go home and thus places the care of the baby in the hands of the parent(s). Ramsay *et al*. (1997) in a study of 9712 babies compared clinical outcomes in babies who had either one or two neonatal examinations. They concluded that there was no clinical difference in the detection and management of abnormalities between the two groups. As maternity units have adopted this policy of one examination (irrespective of the length of hospital stay), it is important to ensure that the opportunity is not missed to provide advice and support for the new family unit.

Role of the examination as a screening tool

Routine examination of the neonate is accepted as good practice (Hall 1996), and its value is recognised in terms of addressing parental concerns (Hall 1999;

Box 1.1 The content of the neonatal examination

The examination should include checking the baby's:

- appearance including colour, breathing, behaviour, activity and posture
- head (including fontanelles), face, nose, mouth (including palate), ears, neck and general symmetry of head and facial features; measure and plot head circumference
- eyes; check opacities and red reflex
- neck and clavicles, limbs, hands, feet and digits; assess proportions and symmetry
- heart; check position, heart rate, rhythm and sounds, murmurs and femoral pulse volume
- lungs; check effort, rate and lung sounds
- abdomen; check shape and palpate to identify any organomegaly; also check condition of umbilical cord
- genitalia and anus; check for completeness and patency and undescended testes in males
- spine; inspect and palpate bony structures and check integrity of the skin
- skin; note colour and texture as well as any birthmarks or rashes
- central nervous system; observe tone, behaviour, movements and posture; elicit newborn reflexes only if concerned
- hips; check symmetry of the limbs and skin folds (perform Barlow's and Ortolani's manoeuvres)
- cry; note sound
- weight; measure and plot

Source: Adapted from NICE (2006: 229).

Townsend *et al.* 2004) and providing parents with knowledge about what to expect from their baby (Walker 1999). It is ideally performed around 24 hours of age (Hall and Elliman 2006) or before the baby is 3 days old (UKNSC 2008a).

The examination provides a valuable opportunity for the practitioner to promote health and instil confidence in the new family unit. For this to be accomplished, the examiner must be able to combine a sound understanding of the physical aspects of the examination with an awareness of the many other significant influences that affect the parents' perception of their baby. Parents also need to be treated as individuals; their need for reassurance will be based on their experiences of pregnancy and childbirth.

Following a systematic review of the literature regarding the detection and outcomes of children with congenital heart defects (Knowles *et al.* 2005) it was concluded that current screening detects only half of those affected. Although other screening tests are available, for example pulse oximetry (Mahle *et al.* 2009), the feasibility of their incorporation into routine programmes needs further exploration, in terms of cost-effectiveness and availability.

Neonatal examination also provides an opportunity for detecting congenitally displaced hips, for which early treatment results in complete resolution in most cases (Gerscovich 1997). It has been suggested that the most effective strategy is to screen all neonates using a physical examination and to offer ultrasonography only to those who are considered high risk, for example a family history or breech presentation (Mahan *et al.* 2009). Overall effectiveness, harm and benefits of this examination remain controversial (Dezateux and Rosendahl 2007). Timing of the examination is an issue with approximately 60% of those who screened positive during the first examination being normal by 1 week of age (Townsend *et al.* 2004).

It is difficult to obtain clear evidence about the effectiveness of the examination of the newborn as it is deemed unethical to conduct a randomised controlled trail in which one group of babies do not receive an examination (Townsend *et al.* 2004). Continued evaluation of detection rates at differing times and by different practitioners remains a high priority.

Who should undertake the examination of the newborn?

The person undertaking the examination of the newborn has traditionally been a paediatrician (Lumsden 2002) but following the initial work of Michaelides and her colleagues (1995) opportunities have become available for non-medics to develop their skills in this area. Increasingly midwives and neonatal nurses are undergoing additional programmes of education and supervised practice to enable them to fulfil this role (Mitchell 2003).

In a postal survey (Hayes *et al.* 2003) it was reported that 83% of examinations were being conducted by senior house officers (SHOs) and that, although 2% of all midwives are qualified to undertake the examination, one-third were not practising this skill. Steele (2007) undertook a qualitative study to identify why midwives were not pursuing this aspect of their professional role. A combination of barriers was identified including lack of appreciation of their role; work load and role conflict; lack of equipment; and isolation and lack of support. Another factor that compounds the problem is that the fewer examinations the midwife undertakes the more likely she is to feel that she is losing her skills (McDonald 2008). This lack of confidence is likely to result in the midwife conducting fewer examinations and so the cycle continues. However, where midwives are fulfilling their enhanced role, they also report greater job satisfaction (McDonald 2008; Hutcherson 2010).

It is imperative that midwives work with their managers and the wider multi-professional team to explore robust mechanisms to enable all professionals to develop and maintain their skills.

Examining effectiveness

Midwives who take on the role of examining newborn babies and those leading the service need to know if they are as effective as their medical colleagues. The EMREN study was conducted with the remit of assessing the implications and cost-effectiveness of extending the role of midwives to include the routine examination of the healthy newborn (Townsend *et al.* 2004). It looked at the following features in detail:

- appropriate referrals;
- problems identified in baby's first year of life;
- quality of the examination;
- maternal satisfaction;
- opinions of professionals and mothers about the examination;
- cost-effectiveness.

The EMREN study is summarised below, to enable midwives to regain their confidence and recognise their ability and success as safe and effective practitioners.

Methodology

A range of methods was use to address the aims of the study. A randomised controlled trial of 871 eligible participants was conducted to look at the effectiveness of the examination. The quality of the examination was judged using video recordings of 11 midwives and seven SHOs (a total of 39 examinations were recorded). A data collection proforma was developed and piloted. Four observers, two consultant paediatricians and two senior midwife examiners rated the videos, and these observers were from different hospitals and did not know the staff.

Maternal satisfaction was measured by questionnaire after the examination and again three months later. The opinions of the professionals and women were sought and in-depth interviews were conducted with 10 women, 10 midwives, 10 general practitioners and 10 SHOs. In addition, the different models of care were explored in relation to their cost-effectiveness.

Appropriate referrals

One of the main reasons for conducting the routine examination of the newborn is to screen for health problems and this may result in a referral for a minor or potentially major problem. The aim was to look at how appropriate the referrals had been, rather than the outcome of the referral.

An appropriate referral was defined as one in which there was an indication that the child might be at risk or require further diagnosis, intervention, monitoring or reassurance to parents, and which, if missed, could be detrimental to the child's health. Independent consultant opinion was sought as to whether any of the problems identified in the first year should have been detected at 24 hours.

Data were collected from 826 examinations and some problems or abnormalities were detected in 32% of the sample. Most of these were noted but not referred. More problems were noted by midwives but not referred whereas SHOs tended to note problems only if they were going to be referred. SHOs made 19/418 appropriate referrals to a hospital specialist and midwives made 24/408 appropriate referrals (4.6% and 5.9% respectively). This difference was not statistically significant. Inappropriate referrals were made in 4/418 SHO examinations and 5/408 midwife examinations (0.95% and 1.22% respectively). This difference was not statistically significant.

Problems identified in the first year of life

The study collected data regarding problems picked up at three months and up to a year.

Primary care consultations within the first three months were mainly for minor ailments, coughs, colds and rashes. There were no significant differences in consulting primary care by whether the baby had been examined by an SHO or a midwife. Three of the 14 cardiac problems identified at the time of the three-month follow-up had been detected at the first examination.

For the problems identified by one year it was judged that 11% should have been picked up at the first examination, but the detection of problems did not differ significantly by who examined the baby at 24 hours.

Quality of the examination

Midwives' examinations were judged to be of higher quality than the doctors in terms of both technical and communication skills. It was disappointing, however, that for certain components of the examination neither midwives nor doctors scored highly, particularly for hip screening using Barlow's test. Examiners rarely raised the question of family history and the baby was often not relaxed during the hip examination or when the heart sounds were being auscultated.

Maternal satisfaction

Generally maternal satisfaction was high, with 81% reporting that they were satisfied or very satisfied. However, mothers were more satisfied when a midwife rather than an SHO examined their baby. Midwives were more likely to discuss health-care issues and be able to provide continuity of care. Once these had been accounted for in the analysis there was no difference between the groups, suggesting that undertaking such discussions has the potential to increase maternal satisfaction.

Opinions of professionals, mothers and consumer groups about the examination

Both doctors and midwives valued the examination of the newborn as a useful tool that gave reassurance to parents, although some felt that it had the potential for parents to put too much faith in it. Midwives were most likely to consider the examination an appropriate time to discuss health-care issues. Others, including mothers, had a mixed response to this aspect of the examination, some finding it a useful time to ask additional questions and others not having any issues to raise.

The doctors were comfortable with the idea of and experience of midwives carrying out the examination but felt that there were too many exclusions (in this study just over 50% of babies were eligible for a midwife examination because of exclusions such as instrumental birth, caesarean under general anaesthetic, infection in the mother, weight and gestation exclusions, etc). Doctors felt that they should have experience handling newborn babies but should have more formal teaching, especially in examining hearts, hips, eyes and femoral pulses.

Most midwives welcomed an extension of their role as it increased continuity of care, enhanced their job satisfaction and was felt to be within the scope of normal practice. However, many were concerned about their workload and the competing demands on their time.

Mothers thought that the continuity that midwives could offer was good, plus it offered the possibility of being able to go home sooner. They usually felt happy with whoever did the examination as long as they were competent.

All of the Royal Colleges and consumer group organisations were supportive of midwives performing the newborn examination. They saw that the midwife could provide continuity of care, continue in her role as health educator and communicate easily with the mother. It was felt, however, that the criteria enabling midwives to examine need to be extended to allow more babies to fall within their remit. This should be in tandem with the adoption of clear referral pathways. It was acknowledged that the impact on SHO training would need to be taken into account if more midwives undertook this role.

Costs

It was concluded that if midwives were to examine all babies for whom there were no complications of birth or antenatal history (i.e. about 50% of newborns) there would be savings of about £2 per baby. Overall the economic implications were not huge.

The EMREN study has raised some important issues, with messages for us all in clinical practice, education and research.

Education and competence

In 2004, with a revision in 2008, NHS Quality Improvement Scotland published *Best Practice Statements* in relation to examination of the newborn. These are a comprehensive collection of detailed and auditable standards that not only identify best practice, but also provide a rationale and means of demonstrating that they have been achieved. Each statement is accompanied by a list of challenges, acknowledging that the practitioner usually works in a context in which they are performing multiple tasks and roles.

The statements are divided into three sections:

1. the where, when, what and by whom of the routine examination of the newborn;
2. post-registration training for registered maternity care professionals undertaking the routine examination of the newborn;
3. the actual examination of the newborn.

Core competencies for the newborn examiners are outlined in the 2004 version of the statement and provide consistency across higher education institutions (see Box 1.2). The 2008 version has the added value of a downloadable

Box 1.2 Core competencies: NHS Quality Improvement Scotland

The Scottish Routine Examination of the Newborn Course Core Competencies for Maternity Care Professionals Conducting the Routine Examination of the Newborn

1.0   Cognitive

1.1   Interprets the significance of the maternal, family and perinatal histories, in relation to the examination of the newborn

1.2   Knows how to refer, and demonstrates this by selecting the correct referral pathway

1.3   Provides accurate information to the key professional(s)

1.4   Generates clear and concise reports

1.5   Generates complete reports contemporaneously

2.0   Psychomotor

2.1   Adapts the environment to ensure adequate lighting and warmth during the examination of the newborn

2.2   Creates an environment that ensures privacy for the parents and the baby during the examination of the newborn

2.3   Adapts the environment to ensure the baby's safety and comfort during the examination of the newborn

2.4   Performs the examination of the newborn using a systematic approach

2.5   Differentiates between normal and abnormal/unexpected findings during the examination

2.6   Compiles contemporaneous records of the examination

2.7   Identifies the parental needs in relation to information giving during the examination

2.8   Responds to the needs of parents in a respectful and supportive manner

2.9   Explains the procedure for the examination of the newborn to the parents

2.10 Responds effectively to the concerns expressed by parents

2.11 Organises referrals according to the local procedures

2.12 Explains effectively the need for referral to the parents

3.0   Affective

3.1   Explains the findings of the newborn examination clearly and concisely

3.2   Verifies parents' understanding of oral communication relating to the examination of the newborn

Source: NHS Quality Improvement Scotland (2004: 17).

audit tool, enabling practitioners to undertake a comprehensive evaluation of the service they provide.

In 2008, the UK National Screening Committee (NSC) published standards and competencies for the newborn and physical examination. The competencies are divided into six parts and are mapped to the Key Skills Framework (KSF) (see Box 1.3). Each competency is further broken down into *benchmarks*, and examples of knowledge and skills accompany these.

It is therefore expected that programmes of education will include these competency frameworks in their curricula, thus providing consistency and transferability of skills. These competencies should be applied to all professionals who undertake the examination of the newborn, irrespective of professional qualification. These competencies serve as a valuable basis from which to audit practice (see Chapter 8).

Future developments

Members of the Royal Colleges interviewed as part of the EMREN study (Townsend *et al.* 2004) were generally supportive of the concept that training for the examination of the newborn should be part of pre-registration education. The exception was the Royal College of Paediatrics and Child Health, which suggested maintaining specialist training so that a few midwives carry out the examinations.

Box 1.3 Competencies for newborn physical examination (UK NSC 2008)

Newborn and Infant Physical Examination – Standards and Competencies

1. Determines the relationship between antenatal (before birth) and intra-partum (occurring during labour and delivery) events that may impact on the newborn's health status, and subsequent events that may impact on the 6- to 8-week infant
2. Ensures that the environment is conducive to effective and safe examination
3. Facilitates effective informed decision-making
4. Utilises a holistic, systematic approach, to comprehensively examine the neonate/infant effectively and sensitively
5. Records and communicates findings to parents and relevant professionals
6. Maintains and further develops professional competence in examination of the newborn/6- to 8-week infant

Source: UK NSC (2008a).

Respondents in the study by McDonald (2008) also felt that training for the examination of the newborn should be integrated into the current midwifery training. In support of this potentially controversial view, from 2010 the module will be an option for students at Anglia Ruskin University with a possibility when the programme is revalidated in four years that it will form part of every student's education. An online module is also being developed for health visitors carrying out the 6- to 8-week examination.

Summary

There is a range of practitioners who undertake the examination of the newborn, all with a unique and valuable perspective to bring. Initial education and skill development should be supported and underpinned by a comprehensive programme of updates and an audit of practice. This concept is succinctly summarised by Hall and Elliman (2006: 337): 'The professional qualification of the person(s) delivering various aspects of this [screening] programme is less important than the quality of their initial training and continuing training, audit and self monitoring'.

Self-test

1. When is the optimum time to conduct the first examination of the newborn?
2. List three aims of the examination of the newborn.
3. What are the barriers faced by midwives who wish to practice as a neonatal examiner?
4. Why is it important that more non-medics become neonatal examiners?
5. What did the EMREN study show in relation to the rate of appropriate referrals between doctors and midwives?
6. What did the EMREN study show in relation to the satisfaction experienced by women when their baby was examined by either a doctor or a midwife?
7. What did the EMREN study show in relation to members of the Royal Colleges and the educational provision for examination of the newborn?
8. Reflect on the learning outcomes for your local preparation programme. How do they differ from the UK and Scottish outcomes published in 2008?
9. What is the value of core competencies for newborn examiners?
10. Identify three advantages and three disadvantages of including neonatal examiner preparation in pre-registration education programmes.

Activities

Consider the following questions in relation to the service you offer:

Choice

In the realm of health-care provision there is increasing emphasis on offering choice to women. However, this is a difficult concept to put into practice when, in many cases, there are limited choices to offer. For example, are we able to ask women whether they would like their baby examined at home or in hospital? Are there sufficient practitioners in either setting to make this a realistic option? Do we ever ask parents if they would prefer a midwife, neonatal nurse or paediatric SHO to examine their baby? When resources are tight, the choices on offer will be restricted. However, this should not stop us asking questions of our care or looking at small ways in which we can offer some choices – even the choice of carrying out the examination next to the bed or in a more private location or the opportunity for the partner to be present.

Continuity of carer

Being able to build on the information you already have about a family during a neonatal examination is a valuable starting point. Equally important is the opportunity to continue to reinforce issues that were previously discussed in the examination. Practitioners need to explore if there are any opportunities to increase the number of examinations that are performed by a previously known practitioner and to identify and develop models of care that best lend themselves to this approach. Where it is not possible to implement such a model across the service, it might it be worth exploring this approach with vulnerable families in the first instance.

Quality

We constantly need to question and explore the barriers for improving practice. For example, are our examinations opportunistic or are we able to offer parents an approximate time when we will examine their baby? If not why not? What is standing in our way? Is it possible to overcome these obstacles?

Resources

- The Newborn and 6- to 8-week Infant Physical Examination Digital Toolbox has been prepared for the UK National Screening Committee. Designed to collate existing resources, the toolbox contains listings of journal articles, books and reports, CD-ROMs/videos, websites and simulators relevant to the physical examination of the newborn and 6- to 8-week infant. http://hearing.screening.nhs.uk/toolbox/

- NHS Quality Improvement Scotland. (2008). *Best Practice Statement – May 2008. Routine Examination of the Newborn*. This is the second edition of a publication from the NHS in Scotland. The first edition in 2004 outlined a template for a Scottish programme on examination of the newborn and this has been adopted across the country. http://www.nhshealthquality.org/nhsqis/files/20219%20BPS_Newborn%20.pdf; http://www.nhshealth-quality.org/nhsqis/files/Routine%20Examination%20of%20the%20Newborn%20BPS%202008.pdf

- *Newborn and Infant Physical Examination – Standards and Competencies*. The National Screening Committee have now produced standards and competencies that are mapped to the Key Skills Framework and the Skills for Health competencies. These are auditable standards and apply to all who currently practice the newborn examination as well as those in training. http://newbornphysical.screening.nhs.uk/publications

- Townsend *et al*. (2004). Routine examination of the newborn: the EMREN study. Evaluation of an extension of the midwife role including a randomised controlled trial of appropriately trained midwives and paediatric senior house officers. http://www.hta.ac.uk/execsumm/summ814.shtml

- *NHS Newborn and Infant Physical Examination (NIPE) Programme – Care Pathways*. These process maps reflect the NIPE care pathways contained within the national competencies and standards guidance for NIPE. There is one overall process map for the newborn and infant physical examinations together with one for each of the four specialist areas – eyes, heart, hips and testes. http://newbornphysical.screening.nhs.uk/carepathways

- Royal College of Midwives. (2009). Examination of the newborn CD-ROM. http://www.rcm.org.uk/college/resources/bookshop/resources/?entryid10=103119

Chapter 2   In the beginning

- Introduction
- Becoming a mother
- Premature and mature motherhood
- Infertility
- Questions that new parents may ask
- Summary
- Self-test
- Activities
- Resources

Introduction

The aim of this chapter is to set the scene for a comprehensive and sensitive examination of the newborn infant. Each woman's experience of becoming a mother is different and unique to her individual circumstances. The practitioner who examines her baby will be able to provide a woman-centred approach to this important examination if she does so with an appreciation of the factors that may influence the experience of motherhood. Such an understanding will also enable the practitioner to place in context any questions that may be raised by parents. Failure to consider the unique circumstances of individual women and their immediate families could potentially lead to care that is ritualistic. Parents should feel that the practitioner who examines their baby is focused specifically on them.

There are a multitude of variables that will impact on individual women and their experiences that we can only glimpse at in this context. This chapter provides a taster to help you reflect on how each journey into parenthood will be different and that this uniqueness must be reflected in the care that each woman receives. It aims, therefore, to encourage the practitioner to consider:

- factors that may influence a woman's decision to have a baby;
- the implications of premature and mature motherhood;
- the experience of women who have become pregnant through assisted conception;
- questions that new parents may raise.

Scenarios will be used to explore specific issues, focusing on the role of the practitioner undertaking the first examination of the newborn.

Becoming a mother

The average number of babies per woman in the UK is now 1.98 (National Statistics 2009). The decision to embark on the pleasure of parenthood is rarely made immediately before conception but is a culmination of a woman's culture, age, social class, peer pressure and relationship status. Each decision to 'try for a baby' is unique to that individual, and may or may not involve the prospective father. Indeed, it may not have been a conscious decision at all, but the result of lack of knowledge, limited access to effective contraception or a *laissez faire* approach to unprotected sexual intercourse. It is impossible to accurately estimate how many pregnancies are planned; one woman may be reluctant to acknowledge that her now much wanted baby was a mistake and another may not want to admit that she intentionally conceived a baby in less than ideal circumstances. Reproductive decision-making is a complex issue (Christopher 1996).

Having children is central to many women's identity, providing them with a distinct role and structure to their lives (Woollett 1996). Not only does having a baby confer adult identity but also it is an expression of womanhood, being female. It is almost like becoming part of a club in which undergoing childbirth and the experience of bringing up a child are the essential prerequisites of membership. There is a common bond with other mothers, each having been through pregnancy, the birth and sleepless nights. Children also bring the security of a long-term relationship, and the decision to have children may even have been made because of loneliness in a marriage (Jennings 1995).

Occasionally, having a child may be part of a very specific long-term plan. For example, it is a consideration in some families, for example when there is a child with special needs, for parents to have more children than originally intended. This is not in an attempt to make up for the disability but to prevent a sibling with a handicapped brother or sister bearing the sole responsibility for their care when the parents are elderly or infirm. In some rare situations a baby may be conceived with the hope that it can donate cells or tissue to a sick sibling.

For some women there is considerable pressure on them to reproduce because they are in a stable relationship or because they have reached a certain age. Such expectations may be part of a particular culture, which may also dictate not only when parenthood should be considered but also the ideal family size and preferred gender of the children. Each cultural group also has norms and rituals associated with the birth of a new family member. It is essential that the practitioner becomes familiar with the particular customs that pertain to the client groups in her locality, so that they can be anticipated and accommodated with respect.

Premature and mature motherhood

Teenage pregnancy

Britain has the highest percentage of teenage mothers in western Europe, despite a fall in the number of live births to teenage girls in England and Wales, from 41,089 (46.6% of teenage pregnancies) in 1998 to 40,298 (41.7%) in 2007 (Office for National Statistics and Teenage Pregnancy Unit 2009). Consequently this situation has been the target of government policy; hence, teenagers are aware that their pregnancy may be viewed negatively by the professionals who care for them as well as society in general. The practitioner examining the baby of a teenage mother will need to do so with an awareness of the attitudes that this young woman might already have encountered.

Teenage pregnancy is often cyclical between generations, with daughters of teen mothers going on to have teenage pregnancies (Richter *et al.* 2006). The probability of a teenage pregnancy occurring is also increasing because the age of maturity and first sexual encounter is declining in females. There is a tendency for teenagers to think that it will not happen to them. In a survey of 3820 schoolchildren in England aged from 13 to 16 years, one-quarter (26%) of respondents were sexually experienced and 45% of those did not use contraception (Wallace *et al.* 2007).

Having a baby below the age of 20 years has been linked with poor outcomes such as increased perinatal morbidity and welfare dependency. One study has concluded that teenage pregnancy increases the risk of adverse birth outcomes such as premature birth, low birth weight and neonatal mortality independent of known confounders such as low socioeconomic status and lack of antenatal care (Chen *et al.* 2007). Other variables such as overcrowding and social class are also predictive of a poor perinatal outcome.

Teenage pregnancies are sometimes carefully planned with positive outcomes (Quinlivan 2004). It may be a means of escaping an unhappy home (Roch *et al.* 1990), creating someone who will give them unconditional love (Alcock 1992) or enhancing low self-esteem by achieving something of worth (Chaplin and McDiarmid 1992). It may also be the conscious decision of two committed individuals and should not be viewed as a childish error of judgement.

The young mother will undoubtedly have experienced negative attitudes towards her at some stage during her pregnancy. The practitioner examining her baby can help boost her confidence and morale by focusing on the positive aspects of her achievement. It is also an opportunity to raise issues such as immunisation or how to recognise when the baby is unwell as part of the natural flow of the examination, rather than in a preaching or superior manner.

Mature motherhood

The age at which women decide to commence child rearing is increasing in developed countries; for example in 2006 the mean age for giving birth was 29.2 years, compared with 28.6 years in 2001 (The Information Centre 2009). Increasing maternal age has long been associated with poor obstetric outcomes. In a prospective multicentre investigation of 36,056 women (the FASTER trial) multivariable logistic regression analysis was used to assess the effect of age on outcomes after adjusting for race, parity, body mass index, education, marital status, smoking, medical history, use of assisted conception, and patient's study site. It concluded that older women were more likely to experience miscarriage, gestational diabetes, placenta praevia and caesarean section. Women aged over 40 years also had an increased risk of placental abruption, low birth weight and perinatal mortality (Cleary-Goldman *et al.* 2005). Women who are over the age of 35 years when they conceive have an increased risk of having a baby with Down's syndrome, and the issues surrounding antenatal screening for this condition are discussed in Chapter 3.

A woman who waits until she is older may feel emotionally and physically prepared for parenthood. If she is employed, she is more likely to have reached a more senior position within her chosen career and therefore be more financially secure. She may also have taken the opportunity to access and implement pre-conceptual advice, such as taking folic acid, reducing her alcohol intake and stopping smoking.

This rosy picture is idealistic and rather naive. Assuming that the woman is employed, she is more likely to feel socially isolated when she does give up work and be concerned that she is losing her place on her chosen career ladder. If she has always been at work during the day she may have had little opportunity to develop close links and friendships with her neighbours. It may be difficult for her to combine motherhood with employment in the future because of shift patterns or inadequate childcare facilities, and this may be a source of anxiety, especially if her wage is relied on. Particularly in areas of high male unemployment, many women are the sole wage earners, sometimes combining more than one job in order to pay the bills.

Women can face financial hardship at any age and may approach the practitioner who examines their baby for information regarding the benefits that they are entitled to. In such cases, women should be offered current, high-quality written information in addition to referral to the appropriate member of the multidisciplinary health-care team.

Avoiding stereotypes

We have taken a glance at some of the issues that mothers may face depending on their age. It is important to explore how this knowledge might influence the care that you give when undertaking the first examination of the newborn. Consider the following scenario:

> You are caring for two women whose babies need their first neonatal examination before they go home from hospital. One mother is 15 years of age and the other is 40. Before you undertake the examinations you take a moment to reflect on the assumptions and stereotypes that you have of these women. How can you ensure that you provide appropriate care?

To illustrate the fact that professionals often categorise certain types of women, some of the common stereotypes that are attributed to teenage mothers are listed below. Of course, such descriptions could also be applied to the 40-year-old mother. The fact is that, unless we know, we should not assume.

- *Limited knowledge regarding baby care*. It is very easy to assume that because one mother is young she has no experience caring for young babies. It could actually be the case that she has played a large part in the care of younger siblings and is confident and adept and looking forward to caring for her own child.
- *Unplanned pregnancy*. On the contrary, this may have been a much wanted and intended pregnancy.
- *Unsupported, lonely and isolated*. This young woman may have a very close network of friends and family who will be involved in the care and support of this new family. Many families make sacrifices to ensure that new babies have the latest equipment and clothes that they need.

Of course, in reality, all of the above descriptions of the teenage mother may have been applicable. To elucidate the facts about any new mother and therefore provide appropriate care the practitioner should ask each mother the following questions:

- What experience does she have of young babies?
- How does she feel about the thought of taking the baby home?
- What support will she have in the first few days at home?
- Does she have any worries about caring for the baby?

These need not be direct questions, but part of the conversation between the mother and practitioner during the baby's examination.

We have considered how some women choose to delay motherhood; however, for some women this may have been involuntary. The baby that you examine may have taken many years of investigations or painful treatments to achieve.

Infertility

Childbearing has been described as a phase in the life cycle of the family, preceded by the 'couple phase' and followed by a number of new phases including 'toddler phase' and so on (Raphael-Leff 1991). It is therefore suggested that this is the usual course of events, the natural progression from finding security in a relationship. Childlessness has a negative image and often leads women to become stigmatised irrespective of whether or not it is a chosen status. Some women will therefore go to their physical, psychological and financial limits in order to become a mother.

Although the NHS will provide basic fertility testing free of charge, and some areas provide free *in vitro* fertilisation (IVF), there remains some inequality in access to treatment for infertility. Access criteria vary from area to area and often include normal body mass index, no other children living with at home, no previous sterilisation and no women over 39 years [Human Fertilisation and Embryology Authority (HFEA) 2009]. The National Institute for Health and Clinical Excellence (2004) has produced evidence-based guidelines outlining the ideal parameters for successful assisted conception. The result is that many couples pay for treatment, which may amount to thousands of pounds. The success rates for the many techniques that are used to treat infertile couples vary from centre to centre and between methods (HFEA 2009). Success is also influenced by factors such as the cause of infertility, age (particularly the age of the oocyte), sperm and embryo quality, previous obstetric history and pre-existing morbidity. It has been reported that a Spanish woman conceived her first pregnancy aged 67 years through IVF (BBC 2006). She gave birth to twin boys by caesarean section but sadly she died two years later (BBC 2009).

It may not be evident from examination of the woman's case notes whether or not she has undergone investigations or treatment for infertility, especially if donated gametes have been used and the couple wish to keep this a secret. This is entirely their right under the Human Fertilisation and Embryology Act 2008. The practitioner examining the baby must not assume, therefore, that the baby's parents are its biological ones (this may also apply if the baby has a surrogate birth mother). If, however, the mother does disclose having received fertility treatment and this is recorded in her case notes, some of the abbreviations shown in Table 2.1 may be documented.

After the birth, it is a possibility that the mother may feel quite detached from or even indifferent to her new baby, despite her long wait. This is difficult for both her and her partner to cope with, especially when everyone else is so pleased and relieved at the successful outcome. Women will benefit from the gentle reassurance that this is a common reaction following childbirth, and that it sometimes takes time for mother and baby to form a strong bond. There is no evidence to suggest that children conceived through reproductive technologies differ in their levels of psychological adjustment (Shelton *et al.* 2009).

TABLE 2.1 Methods of assisted conception

Type	Description
IVF (*in vitro* fertilisation)	Collected eggs are mixed with semen in the laboratory for 48 hours. Only fertilised oocytes are replaced transcervically into the uterus
ICSI (intracytoplasmic sperm injection)	Prepared sperm injected directly into the oocyte in the laboratory and replaced into the uterus after 48 hours
GIFT (gamete intrafallopian transfer)	Oocytes are replaced with prepared sperm directly into the fallopian tube 36 hours after their recovery
Oocyte donation	Donor oocyte with partner's prepared sperm
IUI (intrauterine insemination)	Seminal fluid deposited directly into the uterine cavity around the time of ovulation
DI (donor insemination)	Donor sperm used to fertilise maternal oocyte
Embryo donation	Embryos resulting from IVF of donor egg with donor sperm and surplus to biological parents' needs

Consider your response to a parent who expresses concern about the effects of infertility treatment on the newborn baby.

The mother whose baby was conceived through the application of reproductive technology may have concerns about the effect of the drugs that she was given to maintain her pregnancy. Such worries are not entirely unfounded in view of the devastating effects of such drugs as diethylstilbestrol, which was used to prevent recurrent miscarriage and led to cases of genital cancer in babies exposed *in utero*, and thalidomide, which was used to treat nausea and vomiting in pregnancy and was held responsible for many severe limb defects.

There is some apprehension regarding children born through intracytoplasmic sperm injection (ICSI) as there is greater manipulation of the oocyte. In a large multicentre prospective study (Katalinic *et al.* 2004) it was concluded that children who are born after ICSI have an increased risk (odds ratio 1.24) of a major congenital malformation compared with those conceived naturally. This small increase is likely to be linked to the parental problems that led to the infertility but a procedural risk cannot be excluded. In a population-based cohort study (Romundstad *et al*. 2008), although there was a greater incidence of low birth weight, smallness for gestational age, prematurity and perinatal death in babies born after assisted conception, when compared with their siblings these findings were insignificant. This again led the authors to conclude that the problems were attributable to factors related to the infertility, not the treatment. We wait with trepidation for evidence of further sequalae of assisted conception in the subsequent children.

For the professional who examines the newborn infant, it is impossible to predict or detect whether or not this baby will have an increased risk of morbidity in future life as a result of infertility treatment. Increasingly, the embryos resulting from IVF will undergo pre-implantation diagnosis (PID), and thus their chromosomal status will be confirmed before being returned to the mother. However, it would be inappropriate to state categorically that this baby will not develop problems in the future (see Chapter 7).

Questions that new parents may ask

Having successfully given birth, the new mother will face many decisions and challenges ahead. She may turn to the practitioner for advice and guidance during this emotional time, and although you will not have all the answers it will be useful to consider some of the issues that could arise so that you can deal with them sensitively. The first thing you must ask yourself is: 'Am I the most appropriate person to answer this question?'

This is particularly relevant if you are not the practitioner with continuing responsibility for that woman. In such circumstances, although you might have the knowledge to provide an answer, some questions should be directed to the midwife who is assigned to the care of that woman. For issues such as breastfeeding, for example, it may be the case that a variety of options have been tried or are planned. Without precise knowledge of previous discussions the practitioner may cause confusion. It may, however, be appropriate to give general advice about future care, but again the woman's midwife should be informed of any concerns that may have been highlighted.

As you gain experience in the examination of babies, a pattern of frequent questions may emerge for your particular client group. Questions such as entitlement to benefits or the presence of local postnatal groups will need to be fielded with reference to the maternity services in your area. These are simple questions to answer, but some questions require more thought. There are a multitude of potential questions, but to help you consider the issues that the new mother may face and how you as a practitioner might handle them we shall explore one question in detail, that of employment.

Employment

For women who have achieved a successful career it is can be difficult for them to fulfil the roles of both a full-time mother and a full-time worker. There can be a conflict of interests; returning to work after the birth of a child enables the woman to develop her skills, communicate with other adults and be financially independent, but it also requires her to become 'superwoman' and juggle many responsibilities at the same time. Although many women are fortunate and share their commitments in a balanced relationship, many more do not and they often have to take time off work when the child is sick or to meet other, numerous responsibilities.

Women who, because of either financial necessity or personal choice, decide to return to work, no matter how definite that decision was, often suffer feelings of guilt. The new mother, overwhelmed by a myriad of emotions in the first few days after the birth, will be susceptible to the views and flippant statements of the professionals she meets.

Consider how a new mother might perceive the innocent questioning of the professional examining her baby when asked, 'Do you work?'

The professional examining the baby may just be trying to make conversation, spurred by the fact that the parent's occupation was noted during close review of the case notes. Whether or not mothers should work is an extremely emotive issue. Many women simply do not have the choice and have to work in order to pay the bills. Others have chosen to stop working and stay at home while the children are young and they are able to 'happily relinquish ambition' (Hampshire 1984).

Many more women return to work on either a full-time or a part-time basis and will need support to minimise the associated guilt feeling they will inevitably experience.

Before the Second World War much attention was focused on the adverse effects of the institutionalisation of children and much of this work fuelled the theory of maternal separation and maternal instinct that became central to the work of Bowlby (1953). This considered opinion took the stance that it was indeed dangerous and stressful for children to be separated from their mothers and that mothers should not work but should stay at home caring for and nurturing their children. We now know that this is not the case and that as long as children have caring and consistent mother substitutes they will not usually come to any emotional harm (Hilton 1991). Despite this knowledge, it is often the former deprivation theory that remains deep-seated in our culture and society. This means that not only do women feel guilty if they work, but also family members, friends and colleagues have something to say on the matter (especially if they themselves stopped working after the birth of their children). There is some evidence to suggest that children whose mothers work part-time or full-time are more likely to adopt unhealthy lifestyles in terms of lack of exercise and dietary habits (Hawkins *et al.* 2009) but this is not a foregone conclusion.

As with all of these situations the converse is also true. Some women who do give up work are made to feel by their career-minded acquaintances that they are missing out on companionship, stimulation and, of course, money by staying at home. The role of the professional at these times of complex uncertainty and guilt is to be the neutral sounding board, enabling women to explore their own feelings without being judged or interrogated. At the end of the day they will need to make a decision that is right for them, not for us.

Consider how would you respond to a mother who asked you, 'When is the best time to return to work?'

This is a difficult question to answer and is of course linked to all the emotional guilt that relates to the previous scenario. There is, however, some useful ground that can be covered in response. For example, if the woman is breastfeeding you can outline ways in which feeding can be maintained even after returning to full-time employment, and you can encourage her to seek the advice of a local breastfeeding advisor, if there is one. In addition, there are many sources of further information such as community midwives, health visitors, La Leche League and the National Childbirth Trust (see Appendix 1).

It is useful to find out what plans she has and fill in any relevant details, such as 'yes, the baby might be sleeping through the night by then' or 'the baby will have had all injections by then', etc. Other useful suggestions might be to encourage her to take a day's annual leave each week for a while so that she becomes used to the new situation gradually. Health visitors often know of local childminders who can be recommended or the facilities that are available further afield. Whatever the woman is planning on doing it must be right for her, but she may ask you what you did when your children were young, if you have any. Even though there are certain stages at which it may be less traumatic for the mother to return to work, it will always be a source of anxiety and grief. This can be minimised by the professional who does not seek to impose rigid strategies but who listens to each individual and their unique social circumstances.

Some of the issues that new parents face have been considered along with the possible responses of the practitioner. No two women or their babies will be the same.

Consider this next account and reflect on how even women with very straightforward social and obstetric histories may face dilemmas when embarking on motherhood.

A personal account

I have always wanted children. When asked as a child what I wanted to be when I grew up, I would fervently retort, 'a mummy of course'. One might suppose that this was a consequence of my upbringing, the environment in which I grew up; however, this viewpoint does not hold water when one considers my sister's reply to the same question: 'I'm going to be the Prime Minister'. I hope you don't think I am some sort of sissy or something, wanting to be a mummy for as long as I can remember, but it is the one thing in my life I never doubted for a second I could do. Even when my sister was undergoing investigations for infertility. Five years my senior, my sister was undergoing dye tests and hormone level measurements when I was ready to start trying for our first baby.

I was in a dilemma. Should I wait until she became pregnant before I tried, because I did not want her to go through the added trauma of seeing me pregnant when she wanted to be? How long would it take? What if she could not have children – I'm sure she would not have wanted me to remain childless too. We decided to go ahead and try for our baby and I conceived straight away. My sister was the first to know and of course she was absolutely delighted, never once making me feel guilty. I never knew how she felt when we were not together.

We laugh now. Her daughter is the same age as my second child – she successfully conceived through IVF. She laughs at the many years of messing about with the whole range of contraceptives available, never knowing what a waste of time they were for her. I'm thankful I made the decision I did.

Summary

It is with appreciation of the preceding events, dilemmas and expectations that the practitioner examines the newborn infant. Although not all of the information may be available, it is important not to jump to conclusions for they are likely to be inaccurate. This is difficult to avoid as everyone uses assumptions to help them interact with people they have never met (Green *et al.* 1990). However, generalisations apply to very few people, so it is more appropriate to verify details that are pertinent to the examination with the mother and use observational and listening skills to complement understanding of the wider context. The range of variables that influence the newborn's environment is vast and their combination covers an even greater range. They will all have an impact on the future life and opportunities of the newborn baby.

The next chapter will focus on normal fetal development and well-being, enabling the practitioner to relate the impact of intrauterine life to the examination of the newborn.

Self-test

1. What is the average age for giving birth in the UK?
2. What are the risks associated with having a baby at either extreme of the age spectrum?
3. What is meant by ICSI and when might this procedure be used?
4. What are your views about maternal employment? Justify your stance.
5. What is meant by pre-implantation diagnosis and when is it used?
6. What factors influence a woman's decision to start a family?
7. Does the use of reproductive technologies pose any risk to the fetus?
8. What is the average number of children per woman in the UK?
9. How old was the world's oldest first-time mother?
10. How would you answer a mother's enquiry into the best time to go back to work?

Activities

- What do you consider to be the advantages and disadvantages of being cared for either by a parent or carer at home or in a childcare facility?
- Find out about the fertility treatment options in your locality. What are the access criteria and payment requirements? Consider the Human Fertilisation and Embryology Act 2008. What are the main features that this legislation has introduced?
- Find out about the local facilities available to teenage mothers in your locality. How can she access multiagency support? What is the rate of teenage pregnancies where you work?

Resources

- *Human Fertilisation and Embryology Act 2008. Explanatory Notes*. http://www.opsi.gov.uk/acts/acts2008/en/ukpgaen_20080022_en_1
- The Human Embryology and Fertility Authority. The regulator overseeing the use of embryos and gametes in fertility treatment and research. http://www.hfea.gov.uk/
- DirectGov. *Financial Support for Parents and Children*. http://www.direct.gov.uk/en/Parents/Moneyandworkentitlements/YourMoney/index.htm
- Department of Health. *Children and Maternity* – http://www.dh.gov.uk/en/Healthcare/Children/index.htm; *Fertility* – http://www.dh.gov.uk/en/Healthcare/Fertility/index.htm
- Every Child Matters, Sure Start Children's Centres. http://www.dcsf.gov.uk/everychildmatters/earlyyears/surestart/surestartchildrenscentres/childrenscentres/
- Parentline Plus. A national charity that works with parents. http://www.parentlineplus.org.uk/

Chapter 3 Fetal development: influential factors

- Introduction
- Fetal development
- Summary
- Self-test
- Activities
- Resources

Introduction

Most pregnancies are free from complications, and the developing fetus grows strong and healthy in preparation for extrauterine life. Some babies are, however, already compromised as a result of hazardous exposure during pregnancy. Before the practitioner begins the examination of the neonate, she will take the essential step of reading the mother's case notes and thus familiarising herself with the antenatal history. It will be in the light of this information that the baby is examined, and the practitioner will need to consider the implications of antenatal events for the mother and baby so that they can be anticipated. Some women may have spent months worrying about something that happened during the pregnancy and may look to the practitioner examining their baby for reassurance.

This chapter will begin with a brief account of normal fetal development to enable the reader to place in context the relevance of potential hazards, such as exposure to rubella, during pregnancy. It will then discuss in more detail the major known antenatal risk factors, giving the practitioner a quick guide to their potential effects. Such knowledge will equip the reader with the ability to reassure and inform parents when they seek advice during the first examination of their baby.

Fetal development

It is important that the practitioner who examines the baby is able to apply knowledge of the stages of fetal development to the individual antenatal history of the baby under examination. Table 3.1 provides a guide to the development of the various systems of the body.

The gestational development of the fetus is extremely relevant to the examination of the newborn, especially if the woman has been worrying about a particular event in her pregnancy, such as an infection. If an abnormality is discovered, it is important to be aware that parents often blame themselves, and that they will make links with episodes from the antenatal period that might be causal in effect. Such concerns need to be listened to carefully and worked through systematically so that they can be put in perspective and usually excluded.

The sections that follow will focus on the most relevant sources of potential fetal compromise and include smoking, alcohol, drug abuse, infection and environmental hazards. Information relating to fetal exposure to these influences is collected during the first consultation between the woman and her midwife or doctor, the 'booking history', and is recorded in her notes (see Table 6.2). Such data may then be updated throughout the antenatal period.

TABLE 3.1 Development of fetal organs and systems

Organ/system	Development
Central nervous system	Spinal cord fusion process by 28 days after conception. Failure results in neural tube defects
Peripheral nervous system	55 days after fertilisation
Digestive system	Stomach, small bowel, appendix, large bowel and rectum differentiated by 16 weeks. Development is so rapid that until 10 weeks' gestation it is accommodated within the uterine cavity. Failure to withdraw back into the abdominal cavity results in either exomphalos or gastroschisis. Sucking and swallowing begin at 8–12 weeks
Cardiovascular system	Primitive heart beating by 4 weeks after conception, valves and central septum of heart by 34 days
Respiratory system	Terminal bronchioles by 22 weeks' gestation, surfactant-producing cells by 23–26 weeks
Urinary system	Producing and passing urine by 10 weeks
Genital system	Sex determined at fertilisation but may not be apparent until 12 weeks. In the male fetus the spermatogonia do not undergo first meiotic division until puberty, whereas in the female fetus this occurs between 8 and 16 weeks' gestation and the maximum number of primordial follicles has been achieved by 16–20 weeks' gestation
Eyes	Almost developed by week 13, although the eyelids remain fused until 24 weeks
Ears	Fully formed and functioning by 20 weeks, although the cartilage remains soft until 36 weeks
Limbs	By week 11 five fingers are distinguishable, and limb movements may also begin at this time. At 17 weeks nails can be identified. Bones begin to ossify at about 10 weeks' gestation
Face	Formed by 12 weeks. Clefts in the nose or palate occur when fusion of the maxillary processes is incomplete

Smoking

Despite the wealth of information regarding the harmful effects on the fetus of smoking in pregnancy, in 2001 approximately 36% of babies were exposed to maternal smoking and 13% were exposed to environmental tobacco smoke (Ward *et al.* 2007). According to Department of Health statistics (Department of Health 2009a) the number of women smoking has fallen, with 17% smoking antenatally in 2005 and 14.4% smoking at birth during 2007/8. However, there are huge variations in smoking rates across regions. There may be many factors that contribute to why women smoke, including addiction to nicotine, habit, lack of support from family, friends and professionals or misconceptions regarding the effects of inhaling tobacco smoke.

The smoke from tobacco contains more than 60 known carcinogens (Hecht 2003) (see Table 3.2). In addition to the dangers that tobacco inhalation poses for all smokers (cancer, respiratory disease, cardiac disease), children exposed to cigarette smoke both before and after birth are also placed at risk of disease and even death. In accordance with the Health Act 2006, all enclosed public areas have been 'smoke free' since July 2007. A summary of the major effects that smoking has on the mother and the fetus is shown in Table 3.3.

The practitioner has the ideal opportunity when examining the baby to offer advice and correct misinformation about this issue. Of course, it is important not to push information on women who are not expressing a desire to alter their smoking habits. However, failure to raise the issue may result in the women interpreting this as a professional being unsure of the facts (Haugland *et al.* 1996) or of not rating the effects of smoking in pregnancy and during their baby's developing years as a cause for concern. It is much more helpful to focus on the benefits of smoking cessation for the woman rather than being judgmental or adopting a moralistic tone.

Simply providing information alone, however, has been evaluated as being ineffective in persuading people to stop smoking (Campion *et al.* 1994). Information should therefore be given in addition to, not instead of, practical support and personal contact with trained professionals, a strategy that has been shown to be more effective (Walsh *et al.* 1997). A systematic review of the effectiveness of smoking cessation programmes in pregnancy (Lumley *et al.* 2008) concluded that the most effective means of getting women to quit was the use of incentives. Overall, cessation strategies are effective in reducing the number of women who smoke and the incidence of low birth weight and prematurity that accompanies the habit. It is therefore important that the

TABLE 3.2 Components of tobacco smoke

Carbon monoxide	Found in cigarette smoke, it binds with haemoglobin, forming carboxyhaemoglobin. It is able to cross the placenta and thus reduces the oxygen-carrying capacity of both the mother's and the fetus's blood
Nicotine	Causes generalised vasoconstriction, which leads to reduced blood flow to the uterus and is therefore another mechanism whereby the oxygen supply to the fetus is reduced
Other chemicals	Acetone, ammonia, butane, cadmium, formaldehyde, hydrogen cyanide, methanol, naphthalene, radon, tar

TABLE 3.3 A summary of the major effects of smoking on the fetus and mother

Effect	Reference
Low birth weight (lbw)	In a retrospective cohort study by Ward *et al.* (2007) (*n* = 18,297), maternal smoking resulted in an adjusted OR of 1.92 for lbw with a CI of 122–171 g. See also USDHHS (1990); Myhra *et al.* (1992); Bardy *et al.* (1993); Cnattingius and Haglund (1997); Robinson *et al.* (2000)
Increased incidence of glue ear	In a study of 32,077 children Håberg *et al.* (2010) found that the relative risk for acute otitis media at 0–6 months when exposed to maternal smoking in pregnancy was 1.34. There was an association until the child reached the age of 1 year. See also Gillies and Wakefield (1993); Strachan and Cook (1998)
Increased fetal, neonatal and perinatal mortality rates	In a cohort of 222 babies who died from sudden infant death syndrome Schellscheidt *et al.* (1997) found an increased risk of prenatal smoking of 2.4 for moderate smokers (1–10/day) and 7.2 for heavy smokers (more than 10/day). See also Haglund and Cnattingius (1990); USDHHS (1990)
Increased risk of asthma	In a cross-sectional study of 13,513 children aged 5–13 years in Puerto Rico Goodwin *et al.* (2009) found that prenatal smoking was associated with increased odds of asthma. See also Neuspiel *et al.* (1989); Weitzman *et al.* (1990)
Reduced milk supply (mother)	In the study by Vio *et al.* (1991) 10 smoking and 10 non-smoking mothers' supplies of breast milk were compared and non-smokers were found to have significantly greater breast milk volume

CI, confidence interval; OR, odds ratio.

practitioner examining the baby is aware of local support groups, resources and initiatives that the woman and her family can access.

It could be argued that, even if women do not make any changes as a result of information that they receive, they still have a right to that information in order to make an informed choice about their health behaviour. A useful model of change, developed by Prochaska and DiClemente (1983), identifies six possible stages that the individual might go through when considering stopping smoking. These are pre-contemplation, contemplation, preparation, action, maintenance and relapse. It is suggested that individuals need to go through each stage of the process to achieve successful 'maintenance', and that, even if relapse into smoking occurs repeatedly, each time they attempt to quit smoking they are more likely to succeed. The practitioner examining the newborn baby can reassure a mother who expresses concern at having already relapsed that this happens to most smokers attempting to stop, but that they are now one step nearer to becoming a non-smoker in the future.

Even if the woman is a non-smoker it is important to discuss the risks associated with passive smoking as there may be family members who need a subtle reminder not to smoke in the same room as the baby. A study by Geary *et al.* (1997) demonstrated that over 50% of women did not receive information with respect to passive smoking. Many women are grateful for the extra ammunition to their request that visitors do not smoke near their baby by being able to say, 'They said at the hospital that babies who live in smoky environments are at increased risk of chest infections or even cot death', which is much more effective than saying, 'I'd rather you didn't'.

Consider the following scenario in which the practitioner examining the newborn baby has an ideal opportunity to correct misinformation:

> I was told that my baby would be small if I continued to smoke during my pregnancy, but he is bigger than my friend's baby, and she never smoked.

You may think that there is little point in discussing smoking issues with a mother who already has safe delivery of her 4-kg baby. However, if she raises the issue it is an opportunity to find out what she knows about the effects of smoking on children. The size of the baby is not always the most helpful argument for health professionals to use, as women can always quote examples similar to the above scenario. The fact is that babies of women who smoke will be on average 200 g lighter and 10 mm shorter than babies whose mothers did not smoke (Bardy *et al.* 1993) – not attributes that most parents would wish to be responsible for.

The woman in the above scenario is letting you know that she is a smoker, and it is therefore appropriate that you inform her of the risks associated with passive smoking, giving her practical advice in a non-judgmental way. It would be inappropriate to be prescriptive and make paternalistic statements about her smoking behaviour. She needs to know that if she makes the decision to try to stop smoking there are many resources available to her, but that in the meantime a positive step she can take now is to smoke outside or in a separate room from the baby. You could plant the seed that perhaps she might not want her child as she grows up to copy her and become a smoker. The key is not to force further information on her but to take your cues from how receptive she is to each aspect.

Alcohol

The Food Standards Agency recommends that women abstain from drinking alcohol throughout pregnancy; however, when women do continue to drink, consumption should not exceed one to two measures once or twice a week (FSA 2008). It is likely that there will continue to be much controversy and debate over establishing what is a safe level of alcohol consumption during pregnancy.

It is known, however, that a moderate consumption of alcohol during pregnancy is linked to a reduction in birth weight. One study (Kesmodel *et al.* 2002) found an increasing risk of stillbirth with increasing moderate alcohol consumption. Binge drinking is known to increase the risk of premature birth (Royal College of Obstetricians and Gynaecologists 2006a) and a consistently high consumption of alcohol is linked to a series of characteristics that together are known as fetal alcohol syndrome (FAS). This syndrome was first described by Jones and Smith in 1973.

FAS affects 1 in 600 live births and is the third most common cause of mental retardation (Seidel *et al.* 1997). It comprises some or all of the following clinical features:

- microcephaly;
- small eyes;
- hearing disorders;
- large ears;
- shallow philtrum;
- intrauterine growth retardation;
- thin upper lip;
- congenital abnormalities, such as cleft lip/palate, heart defects;
- mental retardation.

Affected babies may show signs of alcohol withdrawal at birth and may therefore be irritable and jittery, have feeding problems and emit a high-pitched cry. Babies demonstrating such symptoms should be meticulously examined to exclude conditions such as atrial and ventricular septal defects and be referred to a paediatrician for assessment.

There is evidence that alcohol is most teratogenic during organogenesis and development of the nervous system (see Table 3.1) (Armant and Saunders 1996). Kaufman (1997) describes how exposure to alcohol can induce chromosome segregation errors in the ovulated oocyte. Such eggs are unlikely to be fertilised but those that are either result in early miscarriage or, very rarely, proceed to develop into children with severe mental retardation. Alcohol consumption has also been associated with reduced fertility in women (Jensen *et al.* 1998).

Consider the following expression of concern from a new mum:

> I'm really worried. I became pregnant after getting drunk at a party. I don't normally drink but I'm worried I may have harmed the baby.

The research states that for someone who is well nourished and is not a heavy drinker normally getting drunk in early pregnancy is unlikely to have caused the baby any problems (Tolo and Little 1993). It would be particularly valuable to explain to her the sort of problems associated with excessive alcohol consumption during pregnancy and systematically show her, for example, that the baby's head is the expected size, that its eyes, ears and lips all appear to be normal. Of course, you cannot tell her that her baby will not develop problems in the future, but you can say that at the moment you do not have any concerns about the baby. If it is appropriate you could perhaps make sure that she is aware of the potential danger of suffocation if she has the baby in bed with her after she has consumed alcohol, especially if, as new parents often are, she is extremely tired. Unsafe sleeping conditions are often implicated in cases of unexpected deaths in infants (Beal and Byard 1995), and the examination of the newborn is an ideal opportunity to inform *all* parents about current perspectives regarding safe sleeping conditions for babies (see Appendix 2)

Drug abuse

In cases in which it is clearly evident from the woman's case notes that she has been abusing drugs during her pregnancy, the baby must be referred to a paediatrician so that the need for medical treatment or long-term care can be assessed. However, not all women disclose their addiction.

The practitioner examining the newborn baby may be alerted to the possibility that the mother has abused drugs during her pregnancy if the baby demonstrates symptoms of withdrawal, called neonatal abstinence syndrome (NAS), including irritability, poor feeding, vomiting, high-pitched cry and tremor. The degree of withdrawal is dependent on the types of drugs and the amount consumed.

Heroin

High doses of heroin taken by the mother are likely to cause the baby severe problems in the perinatal period. The baby will demonstrate the symptoms of withdrawal mentioned above and is also more likely to be of low birth weight (Alroomi 1988). It is important to raise the issue that babies whose mothers are heroin addicts should not be given naloxone at the birth, as this could precipitate severe withdrawal. Therefore, for babies exhibiting symptoms of withdrawal, administration of naloxone at birth should be excluded as a precipitating factor.

Researchers have had difficulty identifying the particular effects of heroin abuse during pregnancy because it is invariably used in conjunction with tobacco and alcohol, and the mother often has a poor nutritional status; these are factors that are known to have negative sequelae for the unborn child.

As the number of women who abuse drugs in pregnancy rises, the expertise of the agencies caring for them also increases. In areas where substance misuse is particularly prevalent, teams of professionals work together to offer support and treatment for pregnant women (McIver 2007). A Cochrane review of home visits during pregnancy versus no visits did not find sufficient evidence to recommend such an intervention (Doggett *et al.* 2005). The baby born to a mother on a low-dose methadone programme may not exhibit any symptoms at all or may have mild symptoms that persist for a few months (Roberton 1996).

A baby that is showing symptoms of opiate withdrawal should be referred to a paediatrician for management of care as long-term follow-up may be indicated. It should be nursed in a quiet environment and be offered small, frequent feeds.

Cocaine

Use of this central nervous system stimulant in pregnancy is linked with shorter body length, reduced head circumference and intrauterine growth retardation associated with placental and uterine vasoconstriction (Polin and Fox 1998). A longitudinal study has shown that children who were exposed to cocaine during the first trimester grew at a slower rate than those who were not exposed (Richardson *et al.* 2007). Those children who were exposed were smaller at 7 and 10 years, but not at 1 or 3 years, demonstrating a persistent effect on growth.

Such effects may be confounded by the fact that cocaine is an appetite suppressant; hence, its users are often of a poor nutritional status (McNamara 1995). The neonate, although not displaying consistent withdrawal patterns, is likely to be irritable and should therefore be nursed in a calm environment (Nora 1990).

Amphetamines

Plessinger (1998) describes the risks of adverse outcomes for the fetus exposed to amphetamines and methamphetamines, including fetal growth retardation and cardiac anomalies. In a study of 5-day-old babies exposed to methamphetamine (Smith *et al.* 2006) antenatal exposure was associated with neurobehavioral patterns of decreased arousal, lethargy and increased stress compared with non-exposure.

Cannabis

In a meta-analysis of over 32,000 women, English *et al.* (1997) concluded that in the amounts typically consumed by pregnant women cannabis does not cause low birth weight. Unlike many other forms of drug abuse, it has not been linked with an increased risk of perinatal mortality (Zuckerman *et al.* 1989). It has been suggested, however, that when cannabis is used with other substances in pregnancy, such as alcohol and tobacco, it can increase the negative consequences for the developing baby (McNamara 1995). The impact of cannabis use on the fetus is unknown but it may be harmful (NICE 2008).

A note on breastfeeding

For practical purposes it should be estimated that approximately one-tenth of the mother's drug intake will be delivered to the baby through the breast milk (Hull and Johnston 1993). It is important, therefore, that any treatment regime takes breastfeeding into account. Evidence suggests that breastfeeding reduces the need for pharmacological treatment for NAS (Abdel-Latif *et al.* 2006) and that breastfeeding should not be stopped abruptly (Malpas and Darlow 1999).

Transplacental infection

Rubella

If a pregnant woman is exposed to primary rubella infection, especially in the first trimester, the baby may be born with one or a number of serious clinical features, including deafness, retinopathy, encephalopathy, deafness or a heart defect. The risk of a congenital abnormality is 80% if the fetus is exposed to infection during the first 12 weeks of pregnancy (Best 2007). The risk gradually reduces with increasing gestation and is negligible after 22 weeks of pregnancy.

Toxoplasmosis

Toxoplasmosis is a parasitic infection caught from cat faeces and contaminated soil, raw or inadequately cooked meat and unpasteurised goats' milk products. It is thought that about half of the population will have been infected without realising it. If toxoplasmosis is contracted during pregnancy, infection could result in blindness or encephalopathy at birth, or the development of chorioretinitis in later life. At 13 weeks' gestation there is a 6% risk of transmission but a 61% risk of serious neonatal consequences, whereas at 36 weeks' gestation the risk of transmission is increased to 72% but there is only a 9% chance of severe damage to the fetus (Montoya and Remington 2008). If maternal infection is confirmed during pregnancy, antibiotic therapy can reduce the risk of the fetus becoming infected.

The practitioner examining the baby known to have been exposed to toxoplasmosis *in utero* must refer it to a paediatrician for follow-up care. Symptoms rarely present before one month of age.

Chicken pox

Chicken pox is caused by the herpes varicella zoster virus (HZV). Maternal primary infection in early pregnancy may lead to serious fetal anomalies in 2% of cases (congenital varicella syndrome), including central nervous system damage and eye deformities, although these are rare. Neonatal morbidity is highest when the mother develops the rash in the week surrounding the birth, and it is associated with a mortality rate of approximately 20% (Sauerbrei and Wutzler 2007). Babies born to infectious mothers should be referred to a paediatrician for possible treatment with acyclovir and/or vaccination.

HIV infection

Highly active antiretroviral therapy (HAART) in pregnancy has reduced the rate of maternal–infant transmission to 1% (Townsend *et al.* 2008). There is no way of testing whether babies of HIV-infected mothers will ultimately develop the virus, for all such babies will have acquired antibodies via the placenta. It is only through long-term follow-up that HIV infection can be ruled out, and it is therefore important that such babies receive paediatric follow-up. Infection cannot be diagnosed until the infant is 18 months old as maternal antibodies may persist until then. Breastfeeding is contraindicated in the developed world, where the risk of transmission outweighs the benefits.

Cytomegalovirus

Cytomegalovirus (CMV) is the most common intrauterine infection, occurring in 0.4–3.4% of all live births (Seidel *et al.* 1997). The virus persists after primary infection and can be reactivated. It is estimated that between 1% and 5% of pregnant women become infected, with an approximately 40% rate of viral transmission to the fetus (McCarthy *et al.* 2009). A wide range of malformations may be caused, including microcephaly, growth retardation and nerve deafness, and 10% will display clinical signs at birth. Although routine antenatal screening is not currently recommended, if infection is confirmed during pregnancy, audiology follow-up may be indicated.

Listeria

The sources of the bacteria responsible for this infection are soft cheeses, unpasteurised milk products and meat products requiring reheating. It may be acquired by the fetus via the placenta or during the birth, and is associated with spontaneous abortion, premature labour and stillbirth (Mylonakis *et al.* 2002). Those infants infected before birth usually present with symptoms of septicaemia soon after birth, and the associated mortality rate is approximately 30%. However, when maternal infection is confirmed, antibiotic therapy may improve the outlook for the fetus. Offensive liquor and placental abscesses may have been noted at the delivery. Infants becoming infected after delivery often present with meningitis (Seidel *et al.* 1997) and have a better prognosis.

Congenital parvovirus B19

This virus lives within red blood cells and can be contracted by close contact with an infected person. When contracted by the mother it may lead to spontaneous abortion or hydrops fetalis in about 1% of those pregnancies that progress. Most maternal infections with this virus do not affect the developing fetus. When infection is confirmed during pregnancy, intrauterine blood transfusion may be indicated to treat fetal anaemia (Jong *et al.* 2006).

Environmental influences

Much has been published regarding the harmful effects on the fetus of various substances that women may be exposed to in pregnancy (Barnes 2007). These range from the organophosphates present in pesticides (Shirangi *et al.* 2009) to the lead in exhaust fumes (Hu *et al.* 2006). The effects on the developing fetus include congenital malformations such as cleft lip and hydrocephaly. World attention has also focused on the immediate and long-term effects of radiation, for example after the Chernobyl disaster, including psychophysical effects (Huizink *et al.* 2008).

However, it is almost impossible to attribute an abnormality to a particular cause. It is not always helpful to identify a source of the problem, such as car pollution, if an individual is powerless to do anything about it. If the practitioner examining the newborn baby is asked to answer concerns about antenatal exposure to environmental hazards during pregnancy, the following two examples can be used.

Anaesthetic gases

According to a meta-analysis (Boivin 1997), anaesthetic gases increased the risk of spontaneous abortion before the introduction of scavenging (the system for the removal of waste gases). In a study examining the work of female veterinary surgeons (Shirangi *et al.* 2008) it was found that those who worked with unscavenged anaesthetic gases for more than 1 hour per week had an increased risk (odds ratio 3.49) of spontaneous abortion.

Electromagnetic fields

A study conducted by Sorahan *et al.* (1999) sought information on the occupation of mothers of 15,041 children who had died of cancer in Great Britain between 1953 and 1981. It concluded that maternal occupational exposure to electromagnetic fields (EMF) was not a risk factor. However, a subsequent study (Li *et al.* 2009) has shown an increased risk (odds ratio 1.5) of certain types of brain cancer in the offspring of women exposed to EMF radiation at work. With the increased use of mobile phones and personal digital assistants (PDAs), this issue is likely to be of concern to pregnant women and new parents.

Diet

We have already considered the potentially harmful effects of eating particular foods during pregnancy in terms of the risk of contracting such infections as listeria and toxoplasmosis. It is also suggested that there are risks to the fetus associated with the consumption of a diet that is nutritionally poor, for example low birth weight (Franko *et al.* 2008) and the prevalence of malnutrition in low-income families is high (NICE 2008). By the time the practitioner examines the newborn baby it will already have been exposed to its mother's diet. Other than recognising a growth-retarded baby or the cherubic features of a baby who has been exposed to a high blood glucose level (see Chapter 7), it might be assumed that there is little need for the examiner to be conversant with dietary influences on fetal development. This is not so. It has been seen how opportunities exist during the examination of the newborn infant to correct misinformation and offer advice when appropriate. Consider the following scenario:

> My friend advised me to take folic acid before I got pregnant but I didn't like the idea of taking drugs during my pregnancy . . . well you hear of such awful things happening to babies because their mums took drugs, don't you? Anyway he's all right, isn't he?

There are a few misconceptions demonstrated here. Folic acid (0.4 mg daily) taken pre-conceptually and up until the twelfth week of pregnancy has been shown to reduce the incidence of neural tube defects by approximately 75% (Medical Research Council 1991). Therefore, all women planning a pregnancy are advised to take folic acid until the second trimester (NICE 2008). The fact that the woman has had a baby who is not affected with a neural tube defect does not mean that she is not at risk. Neural tube defects can develop in babies of women of any age and taking folic acid can reduce the risk of this happening. Folic acid has been tested extensively and is widely used by pregnant women and has not been associated with adverse effects on the developing baby.

Folic acid is inexpensive to purchase and is available on prescription from many family doctors. When explaining to women how to reduce the risks of fetal abnormality it may be useful to add that we often do not know what causes defects to develop. Therefore, when we do know of a course of action that can reduce the risk, we should consider it very carefully. Many women feel extremely guilty and blame themselves if their baby has an abnormality and this is exacerbated when there *might* have been a known preventative course of action.

The prevention of neural tube defects is just one example of how the practitioner can respond positively to women's comments and questions during their baby's examination. Verbal advice, especially when it applies to future decisions or lifestyle changes, should be followed by the appropriate literature:

- follow your spoken word with written information;
- find out what your local resources are.

Summary

It has been shown that the practitioner will need a thorough knowledge of a wide range of issues to be optimally equipped to undertake the first examination of the newborn. Although a comprehensive understanding of the physical aspects of the examination is essential, an ability to answer women's questions effectively is also crucial and has the potential to contribute to the long-term well-being of the family.

When there is evidence or even the suspicion that the mother has a history of alcohol or drug abuse, the practitioner examining the baby must ensure that the relevant support agencies are involved in the care and long-term support of this vulnerable family unit. Children growing up within this environment are more likely to suffer from physical and emotional neglect, the aetiology of which is complex. The mother's addiction may be a symptom of abuse that she herself is being or has been subject to and should not therefore be considered in isolation (McFarlane *et al.* 1996).

Self-test

1. At what gestational age does the fetal spinal cord fuse and what is the relevance of this?
2. What are the effects of nicotine on the circulation and how is this relevant to the developing fetus?
3. What advice would you give to a woman who was exposed to exhaled tobacco smoke throughout her pregnancy?
4. What is the safe limit for alcohol consumption during pregnancy?
5. Describe the features of fetal alcohol syndrome.
6. Why should the baby of a heroin addict not be given naloxone after the birth?
7. Is breastfeeding advised for babies of opiate-dependent mothers? Why?
8. At what gestational age is the fetus at greatest risk of being severely damaged by exposure to rubella?
9. What are the risks to the fetus of being exposed to cytomegalovirus?
10. What is the pre-conceptual advice for women about taking folic acid?

Activities

- Find your local policy on the management of a baby with fetal abstinence syndrome. What is the average length of hospital stay for such babies? Find out which agencies work with drug-dependent mothers and their families.
- Find out what action is taken antenatally if a woman who does not have antibodies to rubella comes into contact with the infection. What is the postnatal action in such cases?
- Find out what information is available for women where you work about what they should and should not eat during pregnancy. When is this information first given to women and how is it reinforced?

Resources

- National Institute for Health and Clinical Excellence. Quitting smoking in pregnancy and following childbirth. http://www.nice.org.uk/guidance/index/jsp
- National Institute for Health and Clinical Excellence. Smoking cessation in pregnancy algorithm. Interventions to use with women during antenatal care and beyond. http://www.nice.org.uk/nicemedia/pdf/PH10SmokingCessationInPregnancyAlgorithm.pdf
- British Nutrition Foundation. Healthy eating. Maternal and infant nutrition. http://www.nutrition.org.uk/healthyliving/lifestages/women
- Royal College of Obstetrics and Gynaecology. Green-top guidelines. *Chicken Pox in Pregnancy* – http://www.rcog.org.uk/womens-health/clinical-guidance/chickenpox-pregnancy-green-top-13; *HIV in Pregnancy, Management* – http://www.rcog.org.uk/womens-health/clinical-guidance/management-hiv-pregnancy-green-top-39; *Genital Herpes in Pregnancy, Management* – http://www.rcog.org.uk/womens-health/clinical-guidance/management-genital-herpes-pregnancy-green-top-30
- Group B Strep Support. Information and advice for women and health professionals about group B strep. http://www.gbss.org.uk/section.php?section_id=10&section=downloads
- Group B Strep Support research papers. http://www.gbss.org.uk/content.php?section_id=14&sub_id=62&content=Research%20Papers
- Food Standards Agency. *Eat Well, Be Well*. http://www.eatwell.gov.uk/asksam/agesandstages/pregnancy/

Chapter 4   **Assessment of fetal well-being**

- Introduction
- Booking history
- Antenatal screening
- Diagnostic testing
- Antenatal care
- Summary
- Self-test
- Activities
- Resources

Introduction

The majority of pregnancies have good outcomes despite exposure to potential hazards along the way. However, 3% of babies have an abnormality at birth (Kumar *et al.* 2004), ranging from an extra digit to a major heart defect. The proportion of babies being born with abnormalities has reduced considerably in recent years. There are many possible reasons for this, including an increased awareness of the many potential risks that babies can be exposed to *in utero*, enabling some to be avoided. In addition, recent advances, such as the ability to discover the genetic profile of the fetus and to visualise the fetus as it is developing, enable parents to make decisions regarding therapeutic abortion if an abnormality is detected.

The general purpose of antenatal care is to:

- monitor the health of the mother and baby;
- educate on health and prepare for the future;
- screen for particular abnormalities.

It could be argued that examination of the newborn is a continuation of this process. It is therefore essential that the practitioner has a clear understanding of the events that have preceded the examination of the neonate.

This chapter will build on the previous chapters, focusing on how fetal well-being is monitored in the antenatal period. It begins with an overview of antenatal care and the importance of the 'booking history'. Particular emphasis is placed on antenatal screening and how that should be followed through when the practitioner examines the baby.

Booking history

The majority of antenatal care takes place in the community with many low-risk women going to hospital only for ultrasonography at the beginning of the pregnancy or to see a doctor if they go beyond the expected date of delivery. The woman who has a positive pregnancy test will usually make an appointment with either her community midwife or her family doctor (GP). This first visit is an opportunity for the management of the pregnancy to be discussed and often features little in the way of clinical examination, although this will vary between individual practitioners. There should be a discussion about the woman's wishes regarding place of birth and the most appropriate model of care to meet her aspirations and clinical needs (NICE 2008).

This is probably the most important encounter that the woman has with her community midwife in the whole pregnancy. Not only is it an opportunity to provide the woman with important information regarding diet, smoking and screening tests, but also it forms the basis of a relationship that will continue after the birth of the baby.

The booking history usually takes place in the community, ideally by 10 weeks of pregnancy (NICE 2008). It comprises taking a family history, medical history, obstetric history, social history, screening test counselling, antenatal examination and health promotion advice. This information is essential for the examination of the neonate and should therefore be carefully read by the practitioner before seeing the baby.

An attempt to examine a baby without any previous knowledge of antenatal events would be like applying a generic screening test without identifying the individual needs of the parents and baby. Of course, it would be possible to examine a baby clinically by going step-by-step through the procedure (see Chapter 6); however, a valuable opportunity to provide client-centred care would be missed. Knowledge of the history of a pregnancy should therefore be seen as essential, not optional. For examples of what the practitioner examining the baby should look for in maternal notes see Table 6.2.

Knowledge of the antenatal history can inform and enrich the examination of the baby. Consider the following scenario:

> A mother aged 40 years decided to have an amniocentesis when she was 16 weeks pregnant because she had a 1 in 100 risk of carrying a baby with Down's syndrome. She had spent several days agonising over whether or not to have the test as she had taken 2 years to conceive and did not want to put her baby at risk. Having decided to have the test she then faced the prospect of waiting 3 weeks for the results. However, the cells taken from her amniotic fluid failed to culture and she was asked if she wanted to repeat the test. She declined on the basis that she could not put her baby at risk again and, also, by this time she had felt the baby move and had seen it several times during ultrasound scans. She therefore spent the rest of her pregnancy wondering if she had made the right decision and hardly daring to hope that her baby would be 'normal'.

The practitioner examining this baby, in the light of the knowledge about the amniocentesis, would be able to take deliberate steps to take the parents carefully through the examination of their baby, explaining exactly how Down's syndrome is identified clinically. This would be appropriate in view of the concerns and anxieties that they had experienced antenatally. Although the same clinical features would have been considered in the examination of a baby of a 25-year-old woman with no family history of Down's syndrome, it would not have been appropriate to overtly demonstrate this aspect of the examination.

It can be seen that previous knowledge of the antenatal history can enable the practitioner to enhance the parents' experience of their baby's examination. However, the practitioner must not be complacent. What may be regarded as a near perfect environment for fetal development, in terms of minimal known risk factors and an uneventful antenatal period, has the potential to result in an unexpected abnormality in the neonate. The practitioner should therefore *anticipate the probable and expect the unexpected.*

Despite the widespread use of antenatal screening for fetal abnormality, many women worry that there might be something wrong with their baby. This has been found to be highest at the beginning and towards the end of the pregnancy and is prevalent in 90% of women (Statham *et al.* 1997). The first examination of the newborn is therefore a milestone whereby this fear of abnormality can be either dissipated or, in some cases, sensitively confirmed.

Antenatal screening

It is at the booking visit that all women, regardless of their previous medical or family history, are asked to consider the various screening tests that are available to them. For some women and their partners the decisions are straightforward. For others, however, this may be the first time that they have even considered the possibility that their developing baby is less than perfect. This could be the first step along a rocky road for the small proportion of women whose test results are not what they hoped for, and it is important that the practitioner who examines the baby once it is born is sensitive to the journey already travelled.

Questions may arise at the first examination of a newborn that require a thorough knowledge of the current research evidence, for example:

> I had a transvaginal scan when I was only 6 weeks pregnant. I am worried that it may have caused the baby damage at such an early age. What do you think?

In responding to such anxieties, the practitioner must present a balanced answer. Parents need to be informed that there is no evidence to suggest that there is any harmful effect from the use of ultrasound in pregnancy, although it has been reported that there may be a link between ultrasound exposure and non-right-handedness, especially in boys (Salvesen and Eik-nes 1999). School performance at age 8–9 years has not been demonstrated to be altered by ultrasound exposure (Salvesen *et al.* 1992). The clinical usefulness of ultrasound must be balanced against the potential, as yet unqualified, risks. Although harmful effects have not been shown, the use of higher intensity ultrasound is increasing and it should continue to be monitored carefully. You may also need to show that you understand how test results are interpreted and the action that might follow:

> My blood test showed that I had a high risk of having a baby with Down's syndrome, but after lots of thought we decided not to have an amniocentesis. Does the baby look normal?

There is evidence that antenatal screening for abnormality provokes anxiety in some women. In a study conducted in Denmark (Jorgensen 1995) women undergoing alpha-fetoprotein (AFP) testing with false-positive results were interviewed at approximately 30 weeks' gestation. In total, 46% (56/123) of women whose results were reclassified as normal following an ultrasound scan described being severely anxious, and for some this anxiety was still present when completing the questionnaire. A systematic review (Green *et al.* 2004) exploring the psychosocial impact of antenatal screening concluded that, although a positive screening result clearly raises anxiety, there is little evidence to suggest that a negative screening result puts a woman's mind at rest.

Although the terms 'screening' and 'testing' are often used synonymously, there is a distinct difference between them. Screening identifies those who are at higher risk of a condition than the general population. Testing identifies if the condition actually does exist. As some diagnostic tests carry risk and cost money they are not applied to all. Hence, screening usually precedes testing, unless a woman is already known to be at increased risk because of her age or family/medical history.

The following section will consider the main antenatal screening tests for fetal abnormality that are currently available. It must be appreciated that not all maternity units will offer the whole range of tests described.

Ultrasound scanning in pregnancy

Ultrasound in pregnancy is an accepted and much valued part of pregnancy for the majority of women. It is viewed as a routine procedure during which the baby is measured and the sex of the baby is identified (or not) and after which a picture is obtained. However, it is seldom presented as the screening test that it is. It is recommended that women receive information about ultrasonography before they have their scan (NICE 2008) so that they understand why they are having it and what it may or may not detect.

Dating scan

Ultrasound is also used to determine gestation, which is crucial for the interpretation of many antenatal screening tests, and it is more accurate than relying on menstrual history alone (Wald *et al.* 1992). The National Institute for Health and Clinical Excellence (2008) recommends that all women are offered a dating scan between 10 weeks and 13 weeks and 6 days of pregnancy and that the crown–rump length (CRL) is used to assess gestational age, or the head circumference if the CRL is greater than 84 mm.

Nuchal translucency

An increased nuchal translucency measurement (depth of fluid at the back of the fetus's neck) is used as a marker in Down's syndrome screening. The optimum time to perform this nuchal translucency scan is between 11 weeks and 13 weeks and 6 days of pregnancy. Therefore the dating scan should ideally be carried out within this time. In a multicentre study at the Harris Birthright Centre and four district general hospitals 20,804 pregnancies were included in nuchal screening at 10–14 weeks' gestation (Snijders *et al.* 1998). It was demonstrated that 80% of affected fetuses with trisomy 21 could be identified using this method with a false-positive rate of 5%. An increased nuchal translucency measurement is also a marker for congenital heart defects (Makrydimas *et al.* 2005).

Anomaly scan

A detailed anomaly scan is offered between 18 weeks and 20 weeks and 6 days of pregnancy. The sensitivity of the scan will vary according to the gestational age at which it is performed, the skill of the ultrasonographer, the position of the fetus and the resolution of the equipment. In a study conducted by Friedberg *et al.* (2009) only 36% of infants with major congenital heart disease were diagnosed antenatally despite 99% having had an ultrasound. The lowest detection rates were found for anomalous pulmonary venous return (0%), transposition of the great arteries (19%) and left obstructive lesions (23%).

For some women, especially those who have had repeated scans during their pregnancy, the fact that their baby was exposed to ultrasound *in utero* will be a source of concern. Consider the following question, which you might be asked when examining a newborn infant:

I needed to have a lot of scans in my pregnancy because I had a low-lying placenta. Do you think this could have been harmful to my baby?

Additional ultrasound markers

As the expertise and experience of the technicians using ultrasonography increase, more markers suggestive of abnormality are being identified. Markers may occur in isolation or in association with other suspicious findings and include choroid plexus cysts, 'double bubble' (a finding suggestive of duodenal atresia), dilated renal pelvis (pyelectasia), fetal nasal bone measurement and tricuspid regurgitation.

Choroid plexus cysts

These are relatively common and are identified in approximately 1% of fetuses scanned in the second trimester of pregnancy (Lopez and Reich 2006). The decision to investigate the karyotype of affected fetuses is not clear-cut. According to information derived from a meta-analysis of over 1400 reported cases of choroid plexus cysts worldwide (Gupta *et al.* 1995), the risk of chromosomal abnormality increases to approximately one in three when combined with the detection of other ultrasound anomalies. Choroid plexus cysts have been associated with trisomy 18 when combined with other markers such as increased nuchal fold, but not when they are the only marker identified (Cheng *et al.* 2006). Risk is not related to the size of the cysts or whether they are unilateral or bilateral.

'Double bubble'

Associated with duodenal obstruction, this ultrasound finding is also associated with chromosomal abnormalities in 25% of cases (Cohen-Overbeek *et al.* 2008). There is also a link with duodenal atresia and cardiac anomalies (Okti-Poki 2005).

Pyelectasis

Dilated renal pelves are detectable using ultrasound and may be indicative of an abnormal urinary tract. In a study by Adra *et al.* (1995), renal pathology was confirmed at birth in 44% of pyelectasis cases identified antenatally, the most common features being ureteropelvic junction obstruction and vesicoureteral reflux. All cases of pyelectasis should be referred to a urologist for evaluation after birth.

Fetal nasal bone measurement

There is evidence that in about 70% of fetuses with trisomy 21 the nasal bone is not visible at the 11- to 13+6-week scan and there is also a relationship between absent nasal bone and increased nuchal translucency thickness (Cicero *et al.* 2005). Measurement of the fetal nasal bone has been suggested to improve the performance of first trimester screening for trisomy 21 (Kagan *et al.* 2009). However, ultrasonographer expertise and difficulty in obtaining an accurate image are limiting factors in the universal use of this marker.

Tricuspid regurgitation

There is a high association between tricuspid regurgitation and trisomy 21, as well as other chromosomal defects (Faiola *et al.* 2005). In a study by Falcon *et al.* (2006) fetal tricuspid regurgitation was observed in 74.0% of trisomy 21 fetuses compared with 6.9% of the chromosomally normal fetuses.

Down's risk screening

Until the early 1990s only women over the age of 35 years were offered screening for Down's syndrome as its incidence is seen to rise dramatically with age. For example, the incidence of Down's syndrome at age 25 years is 1 in 1352 live births, rising to 1 in 167 at age 38 years and being as high as 1 in 30 at age 44 years (Rogers 1997). However, over 70% of babies with Down's syndrome are conceived to mothers who are below 37 years of age. Hence, it is now recommended that all women are offered maternal serum screening for Down's syndrome.

The screening test is usually offered on the basis that the woman accepts that further investigations are normally only offered if her result falls into a high-risk category and this is predetermined at a certain ratio. For example, her individual risk of having a baby with Down's syndrome may come back as 1 in 250. The hospital may have a policy to offer further tests to women who have a risk of 1 in 200 or more. Thus she may spend the rest of her pregnancy knowing that she has a relatively high risk of giving birth to a Down's syndrome child, and her decision to have the screening test has not provided any reassurance but instead created doubt and uncertainty.

Of course, the above situation is only one example of how screening for abnormality can raise more questions than it answers. However, the screening test can provide useful information to women who would previously have fallen into the category for routine amniocentesis because of their age. Such women may have a screening test that yields a very low risk for her as an individual, rather than the blanket risk which could have been cited based on age alone, and she therefore opts not to have an amniocentesis, avoiding the potential risk of miscarriage that this test carries.

The preferred Down's syndrome screening option is first trimester combined (see Table 4.1) as this enables the result to be given during the first trimester of pregnancy (UK NSC 2008b). Other options include integrated testing, serum integrated testing and the quadruple test (see Table 4.1). A range of markers are measured in maternal serum (see Table 4.2) and the results are adjusted according to gestational age and maternal weight. Other factors that are known to affect the interpretation of the results include maternal smoking, ethnic origin and diabetes. These screening tests provide prospective parents with not a definite result, but a calculated 'risk' for that individual pregnancy. For first trimester screening a risk of 1 in 150 is the cut-off and for second trimester screening the cut-off is 1 in 200 (UK NSC 2008b). Women with pregnancies that show a higher individual risk are offered diagnostic testing.

Diagnostic testing

When there is a history of congenital abnormality in a woman's and/or her partner's family, or she has screened as high risk for a current fetal anomaly, some form of diagnostic testing will be offered. The options offered will depend on the gestational age, associated risks and technical skill available.

Chorionic villus sampling

Chorionic villus sampling (CVS) is a diagnostic test that is available in many obstetric units. It can be undertaken from approximately 10 weeks of pregnancy and involves the removal of a small sample of villi from the chorion frondosum, either transcervically or through the abdomen.

Chorionic villus sampling has an associated risk of miscarriage of up to 8.2 per 100, although, as Green and Statham (1993) note, this rate varies depending on maternal age, skill of the operator and reporting bias. This high risk of pregnancy loss is a high price to pay for the benefits of early diagnosis. However, CVS is a valuable test for couples with a family history of genetic abnormality, or for women who are sure that they could not possibly care for a child with a disability or life-threatening illness. As actual tissue is biopsied the results are potentially available within 24 hours of the sample being taken (compared with up to 3 weeks for amniocentesis).

TABLE 4.1 Options for Down's syndrome risk screening

| | Ultrasound scan | | | Maternal venous blood | | | | | |
	Dating	Nuchal	Anomaly	hCG (free)	PAPP-A	hCG (all types)	uE$_3$	AFP	Inhibin A
	1st/2nd	1st	2nd	1st	1st	2nd	2nd	2nd	2nd
1st trimester combined	✓	✓	✓	✓	✓				
Integrated testing	✓	✓	✓		✓	✓	✓	✓	
Serum integrated testing	✓		✓		✓	✓	✓	✓	
Quadruple	✓		✓			✓	✓	✓	✓

AFP, alpha-fetoprotein; hCG, human chorionic gonadotrophin; PAPP-A, pregnancy-associated placental protein A; uE$_3$, unconjugated oestriol.

TABLE 4.2 Maternal serum markers for Down's syndrome

Marker	Risk for Down's syndrome if:
Alpha-fetoprotein (AFP)	Reduced levels
Unconjugated oestriol (uE$_3$)	Reduced levels
Pregnancy-associated placental protein A (PAPP-A)	Reduced levels
Human chorionic gonadotrophin (hCG)	Increased levels

Amniocentesis

Amniocentesis involves the collection of a sample of amniotic fluid from which fetal cells are cultured and abnormalities identified. Performed under ultrasound guidance, a pocket of fluid is identified and approximately 10–20 ml withdrawn. It carries with it the risk of miscarriage in about 1 in 200 pregnancies, although this will vary between individual operators. This risk is calculated against the fact that a definite result can be given as to whether or not a baby is affected by a particular condition, and management can be based on this knowledge.

Unfortunately, because this test relies upon a significant amount of liquor being present, it cannot normally be performed before about 16 weeks' gestation. It also requires the culturing of fetal cells, which takes about 3 weeks. Therefore, should a termination of pregnancy be indicated, it would be taking place at almost 20 weeks of pregnancy, by which time fetal movements have usually been felt, the baby has been seen on the ultrasound screen and the pregnancy is noticeable to outside eyes.

Rothman (1988) describes how getting to know the developing baby through the amniocentesis procedure makes the decision to terminate the pregnancy after an abnormal result very difficult. Women who have had a termination for abnormality in a previous pregnancy may relive their feelings of guilt and sorrow after the birth of their subsequent offspring, and the practitioner needs to be sensitive to this and respectful of that decision.

Cordocentesis

This procedure involves the removal of fetal blood via the umbilical cord during pregnancy. It enables rapid karyotyping and haematological analysis. It is rarely undertaken but may provide vital information in cases such as rhesus isoimmunisation. Blood transfusions can also be given *in utero* via this route. It is associated with a fetal loss of 1% before 24 weeks' gestation and 0.8% after 24 weeks' gestation (Liao *et al.* 2006). It would be the remit of a senior paediatrician to examine any neonate who had been 'at risk' antenatally.

Antenatal care

The schedule of antenatal care has changed in recent years to reflect the individual needs of women. The pattern of care in the United Kingdom was originally set out in the 1929 report from the Ministry of Health and stated that visits should be fortnightly from 28 weeks and weekly from 36 weeks of pregnancy. What in the past was very regimented and concrete is now much more flexible and client centred. This change was initiated by work undertaken by Hall *et al.* (1980), which highlighted the fact that many women with uncomplicated pregnancies were being seen routinely. It is now recommended that, for low-risk pregnancies, primigravida are examined 10 times antenatally and parous women have a schedule of seven antenatal visits (NICE 2008). Each attendance has a specific remit and may include an assessment of:

- fundal height;
- fetal heart rate;
- fetal movements;
- fetal position and presentation;
- urinalysis;
- blood pressure measurement;
- maternal mood.

The purpose of each component of the antenatal examination will now be summarised, enabling the practitioner to appreciate the relevance of such measurements to the examination of the newborn infant.

Fundal height is used to assess fetal growth. Traditionally performed by an experienced practitioner using anatomical landmarks, practitioners are now required to use a tape measure (NICE 2008). The distance from the fundus to the symphysis pubis, when measured in centimetres using a tape measure, is a useful (although imprecise) screening tool for the detection of small for gestational age infants. If the fundal height is 3 cm or more less than expected for the gestational age, fetal growth should be investigated further by means of an ultrasound scan. Measurements are made of head circumference and abdominal girth, from which an estimate of fetal weight can be made. Because the rate of growth of the fetus is different depending on the race, height, weight and parity of the mother, the use of customised growth charts has been advocated (Royal College of Obstetricians and Gynaecologists 2002); this has not been universally adopted and is widely debated (Zhang *et al.* 2007). It is important that the practitioner is alert to the recorded antenatal growth pattern in order to make an accurate diagnosis of the baby's health status at birth. For clinical factors associated with large for gestational age and small for gestational age babies compared with the preterm infant see Chapters 6 and 7.

Fetal heart rate is first identified using ultrasound at approximately 6 weeks of amenorrhoea; thereafter it is detectable via electronic means as soon as the fundus is palpable abdominally. The normal fetal heart rate is between 110 and 160 beats per minute (NICE 2007) and varies during rest, activity, maternal drug therapy, maternal tachycardia and venacaval compression. Occasionally, an abnormal rhythm is detected antenatally and if confirmed this requires specialist referral before the birth. The fetal heart rate is also recorded when a cardiotocography (CTG) is performed.

Fetal movements are a simple measure showing that the fetus has an adequate oxygen supply to exercise its muscles. When reduced fetal movements are reported they are investigated by CTG, which examines not only the fetal heart rate but also the ability of the fetus to respond to an increased demand for oxygen. In a prospective study of 752 pregnancies at or over 35 weeks' gestation, Berbey *et al.* (2001) concluded that when women reported reduced fetal movements this was predictive of abnormal CTG, low Apgar score, meconium-stained liquor and intrapartum fetal distress.

Fetal position is recorded from 36 weeks of pregnancy (NICE 2008). If the baby has been in a particular position antenatally, it may have sequelae for the examination of the newborn. For example, if the baby has been in a posterior position the baby's head may be temporarily elongated, which may be alarming for the parents. A baby who was presenting by the breech may continue to extend its legs for a few days. Although this is perfectly normal, it will test the nappy changing skills of new parents!

Urinalysis is undertaken at each antenatal visit and may detect glycosuria (this may occur in reduced glucose tolerance) or proteinuria (may indicate hypertension or infection).

Blood pressure is also measured at each antenatal visit. If the blood pressure is raised in addition to proteinuria (with or without oedema) the woman is said to have pregnancy-induced hypertension. Subsequently, her baby may be small for gestational age and labour may have been induced before full term. The practitioner examining the baby may therefore need to be prepared to discuss the relevance of this condition to the baby and provide general reassurance.

Maternal mood is assessed at each antenatal visit. If a woman has a low mood during pregnancy she is at increased risk of depression following the birth (Leigh and Milgrom 2008). Any concerns about a woman's emotional well-being observed during the neonatal examination should be referred to her lead carer.

Summary

There are a range of antenatal parameters that the practitioner examining the neonate should be aware of in order to be sensitive to the needs of the mother and her baby. Detailed examination of the booking history details and subsequent antenatal records are an essential component of the examination of the newborn. The next chapter considers the impact of events during labour and childbirth on the health of the neonate.

Self-test

1. What is the difference between antenatal screening and antenatal testing?
2. What sample is taken during chorionic villus sampling?
3. When is fetal head circumference used to assess gestational age?
4. What is an increased nuchal translucency measurement a marker for?
5. What screening combination is the option of choice for Down's syndrome and why?
6. When is the anomaly scan performed?
7. Does routine ultrasonography in pregnancy pose any risk to the developing fetus?
8. What is the schedule of antenatal care for women experiencing their first baby?
9. How is fetal growth estimated during routine antenatal care?
10. When is a 'double bubble' seen during an ultrasound scan?

Activities

- Find out what screening test are available where you work. Are they offered to all women? If not, what are the criteria for the different tests?
- Where is your nearest fetal medicine unit (FMU)? Who might you refer to such a unit? What are the implications for the family of receiving care away from home? How can you ameliorate this impact?
- If you noted that a woman had had high blood pressure during her pregnancy, what might you consider in particular when you examine her baby? Do you use customised growth charts where you work? If so, how is their effectiveness monitored?

Resources

- Fetal Medicine Foundation. Information and resources regarding early diagnosis and screening for fetal abnormalities, for example video lecture by Professor Kypros Nicolaides on first trimester screening for chromosomal abnormalities – http://www.fetalmedicine.com/fmf/online-education/01-11-136-week-scan/; the 11- to 13+6-week scan – http://www.studiolift.com/fetal/site/FMF-English.pdf; the 18- to 23-week scan – http://www.studiolift.com/fetal/site/downloads/18-23%2520weeks%2520scan.pdf
- Healthtalkonline. Videos of women talking about their experiences of antenatal screening. http://www.healthtalkonline.org/Pregnancy_children/Antenatal_Screening
- Healthtalkonline. Videos of women talking about when screening does not detect a condition. Learning after birth that the baby has a condition. http://www.healthtalkonline.org/Pregnancy_children/Antenatal_Screening/Topic/1691/
- National Institute for Health and Clinical Excellence. Antenatal care guideline. http://www.nice.org.uk/nicemedia/pdf/CG62FullGuidelineCorrectedJune2008July2009.pdf
- UK National Screening Committee home page. http://www.screening.nhs.uk/

Chapter 5   **Risks to the fetus during childbirth**

Introduction

We have already considered the various risks that the developing fetus may encounter during the antenatal period and how these have relevance for the examination of the newborn baby (see Chapter 3). However, the perfectly healthy term baby may be affected by events during childbirth. Practitioners should therefore possess a thorough knowledge of labour and birth, the difficulties that can arise in childbirth and their possible consequences for the health of the newborn. The events surrounding the birth will be carefully documented in the mother's records, and these should be scrutinised in advance so that the examination takes into account any increased risk factors associated with a particular birth. It is important that practitioners are fully aware of the events surrounding each labour and birth so that they are able to respond appropriately to parents who may, for a number of reasons, have concerns relating to the birth of their child. Although midwives and neonatal nurses often care for neonates requiring additional care, such as premature infants or those with feeding difficulties, it should be noted that only healthy, full-term neonates should be clinically examined by the midwife or nurse. All other babies should be referred to a medical or advanced nurse practitioner, in line with local policy (see Chapter 7) and professional guidance (Nursing and Midwifery Council 2004).

Having ensured that this particular examination of the newborn falls within the practitioner's remit, the following questions should be borne in mind:

1. Was the pregnancy prolonged?
2. Was the labour induced or accelerated and, if so, why?
3. How long were the fetal membranes ruptured prior to birth?
4. Were there any anomalies of the fetal heart rate during labour?
5. Was the liquor meconium stained?
6. What were the methods of pain relief used during the labour and birth?
7. What was the presenting part of the fetus during labour?
8. What was the mode of birth?
9. Did the baby require any resuscitation at birth?
10. Were any injuries or abnormalities noted at the birth?

This chapter will focus on outlining the relevance of these questions to the health of the baby, enabling the practitioner to conduct a thorough and effective examination.

Prolonged pregnancy

The practitioner examining the newborn baby needs to have an awareness of the current perspectives regarding prolonged pregnancy so that women who question the management of their labour understand the rationale behind it. Such knowledge also helps practitioners put into context some of the problems that they might encounter in the neonate.

Prolonged or post-term pregnancy is defined as more than 42 completed weeks of pregnancy (294 days) (Olesen *et al.* 2003) and is associated with an increased risk of a poor perinatal outcome. For example, Hilder *et al.* (1998) in their analysis of 171,527 notified births found an increase in stillbirth and infant mortality from 0.7 per 1000 ongoing pregnancies at 37 weeks' gestation to 5.8 per 1000 ongoing pregnancies at 43 weeks' gestation, signifying an eightfold increase. A systematic review of trials involving 7984 women (Gülmezoglu *et al.* 2006) concluded that induction of labour at 41 completed weeks of pregnancies resulted in fewer baby deaths than expectant management (watchful waiting), with no deaths in the induction group versus seven in the expectant group. However, it has been argued (Wennerholm *et al.* 2009) that no study with adequate sample size to identify such rare outcomes as perinatal mortality has been published

The aetiology of prolonged pregnancy is complex and is thought to include factors such as congenital abnormalities that interfere with the fetal pituitary–adrenal axis and environmental contributors such as diet and pollution (Shea *et al.* 1998). In a retrospective cohort study (Caughey *et al.* 2009) risk factors associated with a pregnancy lasting longer than 41 weeks included obesity, nulliparity and advancing maternal age.

In terms of morbidity, the outlook for the baby of prolonged gestation is generally good because of many factors such as accurate estimation of gestational age using ultrasonography, early intervention after heart rate anomalies in labour and close monitoring of post-term pregnancies (Campbell 1998). However, in a study conducted by Roach and Rogers (1997), it was found that, although there was no increase in mortality before 42 weeks' gestation in pregnancies being monitored, after 42 weeks there was an increased caesarean section rate and incidence of meconium identified below the vocal cords. The incidence of meconium-stained liquor increases with post-maturity and is associated with non-reassuring cardiotocography (CTG) (Wong *et al.* 2002). This may be considered to be an indication for inducing labour post term in order to avoid meconium aspiration.

The views of women experiencing post-term pregnancy are also an important consideration. A study by Sarker and Hill (1996) associates prolonged pregnancy with a significantly higher level of maternal anxiety antenatally, and this may have an impact on maternal well-being in the postnatal period, which the examiner should be aware of. The management of post-term pregnancy is a careful balance between the risks of post-maturity and the risks associated with induction of labour. The National Institute for Health and Clinical Excellence (2008) recommends that induction of labour is offered between 41 and 42 weeks of pregnancy and that, when pregnancy exceeds 42 weeks, women are closely monitored by twice-weekly CTG and ultrasound estimation of liquor volume.

The post-term infant is generally a baby that feeds well and requires little special attention in the postnatal period. Such babies have characteristically dry skin that may be prone to cracking, and parents can be advised to massage their baby with a neutral vegetable oil, which the baby will enjoy, and to avoid using soap-based products when bathing their baby. They may have long fingernails and are therefore likely to scratch themselves, although extreme caution should be used if attempting to trim them because the nail is usually joined to the very tip of the finger in young babies. The use of special scissors under the control of a clear-sighted adult is recommended.

Induction of labour

The importance of the practitioner exploring this issue with regard to the neonatal examination is twofold:

1. The *rationale* for the induction can be followed through; for example, if labour was induced because the mother had pregnancy-induced hypertension, what has been the effect on the baby?
2. The effect on the fetus of the *method* of induction used can be anticipated.

Labour is induced for a variety of reasons, including post-maturity, large or small for gestational age fetus, diabetes, pregnancy-induced hypertension, prolonged rupture of membranes and individual social circumstances. Babies with specific problems will be managed under the care of a paediatrician.

Induction of labour often involves the administration of oxytocin via an intravenous infusion. There has been some debate regarding a link between its use and the incidence of neonatal jaundice (Woyton *et al.* 1994; Keren *et al.* 2005), although, according to Johnson *et al.* (1984), this effect may be more to do with the large volume of sodium solution received by the mother during its administration. Whatever the aetiology, it would be worth preparing the mother for the possibility of the baby becoming jaundiced in terms of what to look out for in the baby's appearance and its behaviour (see Chapter 6).

The risk of a precipitous birth is also increased after induced labour, especially in multigravid women. The practitioner examining the baby must therefore be diligent to exclude the possibility of a tentorial tear caused by rapid moulding of the fetal skull, although such babies would usually be born in a state of shock.

Prelabour rupture of the membranes

Prelabour rupture of the membranes (PROM) is defined as rupture of the fetal membranes before the onset of labour and occurs in about 10% of all pregnancies; 90% of these are at term (Alexander and Cox 1996). PROM at term is managed by either induction of labour or expectant management if there are no signs of maternal or neonatal morbidity. NICE induction of labour guidelines (NICE 2008) recommend that a woman with PROM should be offered the choice of induction of labour with prostaglandin or expectant management. NICE intrapartum care guidelines (NICE 2007) recommend that PROM should not exceed 96 hours. The definition of prolonged rupture of the membranes varies. It is often defined as when the membranes have been ruptured for 18 hours before the birth as this has been suggested as the time after which neonates are at an increased risk of developing group B streptococci (Oddie and Embleton 2002).

In a systematic review of induction versus expectant management of PROM involving 6814 women (Dare *et al.* 2006), fewer women in the induction group had uterine infection. Although there were fewer admissions to the neonatal unit for babies in the induction group, there were no differences in neonatal sepsis rates between the management options. Women in the induction group were significantly more positive about their care.

The number of vaginal examinations that the woman is likely to have performed on her following PROM has been linked to infection rates. In one study (Ladfors *et al.* 1996) comparing two methods of expectant management of PROM, a protocol of infrequent vaginal examinations was associated with low maternal and fetal infection. This result was echoed in the large multi-centre trial study by Hannah *et al.* (2000a), which found that the number of vaginal examinations was the leading predictor of maternal infection.

In a registry study of 113,568 term infants (Herbst and Kallen 2007) the rate of neonatal sepsis was 1.1% after PROM of 24 hours. Although this rate is low, the practitioner examining the newborn must not be complacent about PROM, especially when working within a unit that manages such cases expectantly. It should be borne in mind that the membranes may have ruptured before labour because of infection. It is the practice in some maternity units to take swabs from the neonate if birth is more than 24 hours after rupture of the membranes, and particularly if maternal infection is verified or the liquor was foul smelling. If swabs have been taken, there must be a system for the follow-up of positive results, and the practitioner should endeavour to establish and record the baby's status. It is also prudent to explain to parents how to recognise the signs and symptoms of infection (Chapter 7) and to inform the relevant personnel in the domiciliary setting of all action taken.

Anomalies of the fetal heart rate in labour

Continuous fetal heart rate monitoring during labour was introduced in the 1970s, before it had been shown to lead to improvements in neonatal outcome. In fact, there is evidence from subsequent randomised controlled trials (Kelso *et al.* 1978; Haverkamp *et al.* 1979; MacDonald *et al.* 1985) that electronic fetal monitoring (EFM) increases the risk of caesarean section and operative vaginal delivery. Although EFM was found to be protective for neonatal seizures, those who did have a seizure did not suffer any long-term damage (MacDonald *et al.* 1985). Despite the availability of systematic reviews of the relevant trials (Enkin *et al.* 1995) and NICE intrapartum guidance (NICE 2007) that does not advocate the use of continuous EFM for low-risk women, its use remains popular on some labour wards.

EFM does detect abnormal fetal heart rate patterns but its specificity is poor. It can show bradycardia, tachycardia, reduced variability and reduced response to stimuli. Many fit and healthy babies, however, have been delivered by emergency caesarean section on the basis of an 'abnormal' fetal heart rate pattern. Unnecessary intervention is less likely to occur if EFM is used in conjunction with fetal blood sampling (FBS) to establish the pH of the fetal blood (Table 5.1) (Lissauer and Steer 1986).

The parents of a baby whose birth was expedited on the basis of such findings may require reassurance from the professional undertaking the first examination of the newborn that their baby has not suffered any long-term damage due to lack of oxygen during the birth. It would be a valuable exercise to take them step by step through the examination, highlighting what you are looking for. It is not possible at this stage to say *categorically* that the baby is neurologically intact, but you can state that you have not identified any cause for concern.

TABLE 5.1 pH of fetal scalp blood

Investigation	Normal	Borderline	Abnormal
Fetal scalp blood pH	7.25	7.20–7.24	7.19 or less

A point to note is that use of internal fetal scalp electrodes to record fetal heart rate patterns has been associated with trauma to the baby's scalp (Akhter 1976), and the practitioner examining the baby should ensure that they observe any puncture site and carefully document the findings.

Meconium-stained liquor

We have already seen that the incidence of meconium-stained liquor increases with maturity. The mature infant is also more likely to make attempts to breathe when depleted of oxygen and therefore is more likely to inhale substances present in the birth canal, such as vernix, blood and meconium. This situation – the hypoxic mature infant surrounded by meconium-stained liquor – increases the possibility that the baby will aspirate meconium. Meconium aspiration may lead to meconium aspiration syndrome (MAS), a potentially fatal condition during which the baby has severe respiratory difficulties and requires admission to a neonatal unit.

Babies who have been exposed to meconium-stained liquor but who are not suspected of having inhaled meconium are observed on the postnatal ward. The respiration rate is recorded hourly for the first 4–6 hours and abnormalities must be reported to a paediatrician. The practitioner should also observe the baby for signs of infection as this has been associated with meconium-stained liquor, especially thick meconium (Piper *et al.* 1998).

Pharmacological pain relief

The impact on the neonate of the pain relief used by the mother in labour will be influenced by the following factors:

- type of drug(s) used;
- dose(s) given;
- route of administration of the drug;
- stage of labour drug administered;
- weight of the baby;
- maturity of the baby.

The therapeutic range of a drug is calculated using the body mass index. The smaller the baby the greater the effect of the drug.

The practitioner examining the baby will need to consider all of the above when reading the woman's labour and birth records to assess how this history may affect the neonate. The effects on the baby of the drugs commonly used in labour will be outlined in the following sections.

Entonox

Entonox (50% nitrous oxide/50% oxygen) is inhaled by the mother. This drug is excreted by the mother's lungs and therefore the amount that enters her bloodstream, and hence crosses the placenta, is negligible.

Narcotic drugs

Pethidine is commonly administered to the mother for pain relief in the first stage of labour, although its effectiveness has been questioned (Olofsson *et al.* 1996) and it is associated with gastrointestinal and respiratory side-effects (British Medical Association and Royal Pharmaceutical Society of Great Britain 2008). This drug is given to the mother by intramuscular injection, is absorbed into her bloodstream and crosses the placenta. The dosage ranges from 50 to 150 mg and it is usually given every 3–4 hours. Pethidine has a half-life of 5 hours in the mother and it is metabolised in the liver, but as the neonatal liver is immature the effects on the neonate are prolonged (Gamsu 1993). It is a narcotic and is associated with neonatal respiratory depression (Mattingly *et al.* 2003). Respiratory depression in the baby can be effectively reversed at birth by administering naloxone intramuscularly in addition to establishing airway patency and oxygenation.

The more insidious effects on the baby of lethargy and the lack of interest in feeding are also of concern, especially in the breastfeeding baby. Breastfeeding can be an emotional issue, and a mother who is experiencing difficulties with a baby who does not appear interested in feeding will need support. The practitioner examining the baby can encourage the mother in the above situation by explaining that the baby's response is likely to be a consequence of the pethidine she received in labour and that it is therefore worth persevering. It must be acknowledged, however, that in the first 24 hours after birth the baby will in fact get an extra dose of pethidine via the mother's breast milk, but that thereafter this effect will decline (Freeborn *et al.* 1980). Morphine is also a narcotic drug used in labour, but less frequently than pethidine.

Epidural

In a study conducted by Lieberman *et al.* (1997) involving 1657 women it was concluded that neonates whose mothers received epidurals in labour were more likely to require treatment with antibiotics. This may be related to the fact that epidural analgesia in labour has been associated with an increase in maternal temperature (Mercier and Benhamou 1997), which may lead to the precautionary measure of admitting the baby to a special care baby unit with suspected infection. The use of epidural analgesia in labour has also been associated with a 1.5- to 2-fold increase in the risk of hyperbilirubinaemia but the cause of the link is unclear (Lieberman and O'Donoghue 2002). In general, however, epidural use in labour is not associated with a poor neonatal outcome and is the preferred method of anaesthesia for caesarean section.

Water birth

In many maternity units a birthing pool is available for women to use for its analgesic effects. There is no evidence of any increased risk to the neonate if the woman labours or gives birth in water (Cluett and Burns 2008). An unusual case of neonatal polycythaemia was reported (Odent 1998) in an infant who remained in a birthing pool for 30 minutes after birth before the cord was cut. When a baby is born on dry land the effect of the air causes the cord to constrict, thereby limiting the amount of blood transfused from the placenta.

Presentation of the fetus in labour

Knowledge of how the fetus presented during labour and its relevance to the clinical examination are required so that the practitioner can reassure parents and look for specific features. The following presentations will be considered:

* occipito-posterior;
* face;
* brow;
* compound;
* breech.

Occipito-posterior

This is a relatively common presentation, affecting approximately 10% of babies (Coates 2003). Moulding of the fetal skull results in a characteristically elongated head, which resolves in a few days.

Face presentation

For vaginal birth to take place this requires the fetus to extend its head and neck. The face is usually very bruised and may have a circular demarcation on it (caused by the pressure of the cervix) if there was any delay in labour.

Brow presentation

This rarely delivers vaginally unless the baby is small and the pelvis large. The characteristic moulding results in an elongated sinciput and occiput, with the top of the head appearing flattened.

Compound presentation

This occurs when a hand or foot lies alongside the head. During the birth the operator may have manipulated the limb over the baby's face resulting in bruising or swelling.

Breech

The breech presents in approximately 3% of all term pregnancies. Following the publication of a large, multicentre randomised controlled trial involving 2088 women (Hannah *et al.* 2000b), most breech babies are delivered by elective caesarean section. The trial concluded that a planned caesarean section resulted in reduced risk of perinatal and neonatal mortality and morbidity compared with vaginal birth. The study design and methods have since been questioned (Banks 2001) but the impact of the trial has given rise to a significant reduction in vaginal breech births. However, a subsequent descriptive study (*n* = 8105) (Goffinet *et al.* 2006) found no difference in perinatal mortality between the two modes of birth and this has led to a cautious endorsement of choice of mode of birth for low-risk women (Royal College of Obstetricians and Gynaecologists 2006b; Society of Obstetricians and Gynecologists of Canada 2009).

Breech babies, if born vaginally, may have bruised and swollen genitals, the appearance of which is distressing for parents. If the baby was an extended breech it will lie in the cot with its legs extended for a few days. Parents should be encouraged to clean and handle the baby as usual (although changing the nappy is quite difficult!) and the baby's unusual position will gradually resolve.

Congenital dislocation of the hips is also a potential complication of babies who have presented by the breech position. In an Australian study of 1127 cases of congenital dislocated hips, the risk associated with breech presentation was estimated to be 2.7% for girls and 0.8% for boys (Chan *et al.* 1997).

The head of the breech baby is characteristically round as there has been a rapid journey through the birth canal with little time for moulding. The shape of the baby's head is a positive outcome of undergoing an unusual birth, which the practitioner might like to comment on during the examination for the benefit of the parents.

Mode of birth

This section will outline the normal neonatal outcomes after instrumental and operative deliveries. It is important to note that a paediatrician is not always present at instrumental and operative deliveries, depending on the indication and type of anaesthesia used. The first examination of the newborn may, therefore, be the first time that the baby is clinically examined, unless there were any indications. One study (Jacob and Pfenninger 1997) found that the use of regional anaesthesia for elective or non-urgent caesarean sections reduced the incidence of vigorous resuscitation (defined as bag and mask ventilation, tracheal intubation and cardiopulmonary resuscitation) to a level similar to that of vaginal birth.

Instrumental delivery is the course of action that follows a complication of pregnancy during labour. The examiner will therefore need to consider the relevance of that complication to the baby's health. If the birth was expedited for prolonged labour, for example, is there an indication for screening the baby for infection? When surveying the mother's notes, the practitioner will need to consider the following points:

* the indication for intervention;
* how long the mother had been in labour before intervention;
* the condition of the baby at birth.

Not all women have the opportunity to talk through the events of their labour and birth with the midwife or doctor who was there. This is especially important when events do not go according to plan. In most cases women will have been sufficiently informed and involved in their care to have a clear understanding of what actually happened and why. There will be some women who, either because of the stress of the moment or through the haze of sedation, do not know exactly what happened at the birth. They may turn to the practitioner examining their baby for an explanation of events. Unless it is *absolutely* clear from the birth records why, for example, a woman needed an emergency forceps delivery, always refer her to either the midwife who was at the birth or her obstetrician. Do not attempt to answer questions that you do not know the answers to, but do ensure that she does have the opportunity to see someone who can answer them.

Some maternity units offer a debriefing service for women after childbirth (Smith and Mitchell 1996), but this is variable. The term 'post-traumatic stress disorder' is increasingly being applied to women's distress after an event in childbirth (Crompton 1996), and it must be acknowledged that women may need information and support to come to terms with events (Allott 1996).

Ventouse and forceps delivery

Ventouse delivery is the preferred method when assisted vaginal birth is required as it results in less maternal morbidity than forceps (Johanson and Menon 1999). The risk of serious injury to the baby is low with either instrument, and a review of operative births in nulliparous women concluded that there were no significant differences in the rates of subdural or cerebral haemorrhage between the two methods (Towner *et al.* 1999). A skilled operator will select the most appropriate method depending on the woman's individual circumstances (Royal College of Obstetricians and Gynaecologists 2005). The neonate may suffer damage to the scalp after a ventouse delivery. The anticipated swelling is referred to as a chignon and may be accompanied by bruising and abrasion. Such trauma will be dependent on whether a soft or a metal cup was used, how many times the cup was reapplied and how many pulls were used, and these factors will themselves be dependent on the protocol of the unit and the skill of the operator. A systematic review of the evidence comparing forceps with ventouse (Johanson and Menon 1999) concluded that, in relation to the baby:

- the vacuum extractor is associated with more cephalhaematomata and retinal haemorrhage (see Chapter 7);
- women worry more about the condition of their baby with the ventouse;
- there is no difference in the number of babies requiring phototherapy;
- there is no difference in re-admission rates between the two instruments.

Caesarean section

The caesarean section rate varies between consultants, units and countries and is divided between those that are conducted in an emergency and those that are elective. The caesarean section rate in England has risen steadily from 9% in 1980 to 24.6% in 2007/8 (The Information Centre 2009). It is important that the practitioner identifies why the caesarean was performed in order to conduct a sensitive and effective examination of the baby.

A complication for the baby after abdominal delivery is laceration during surgery. According to a retrospective review of the neonatal records of 904 caesarean deliveries (Smith *et al.* 1997), the incidence of lacerations was 1.9% ($n = 17$). The incidence was higher in non-vertex presentation (6% compared with 1.4% of vertex) and only one of the 17 lacerations was documented in the maternal notes, possibly indicating that obstetricians had been unaware of this complication. The incidence has since been reported to be as high as 3% (Saraf 2009).

The practitioner examining the baby may discover a laceration during the examination that had previously gone unnoticed. It is important not to attempt to hide such a discovery from the parents, but to explain that this is a complication of caesarean section because of the close proximity of the fetus to the uterine wall. The significance of a laceration to the parents should not be undermined, especially if it is on the baby's face, but most parents can balance this with the relief that their baby's birth was expedited to avoid a much more serious outcome. The obstetrician who conducted the birth should be informed of the laceration and careful records made. Such wounds are usually clean and heal quickly with the aid of a steri-strip. A red scar may persist for some weeks but will eventually fade and become unnoticeable.

Babies born by caesarean section have an increased risk of developing transient tachypnoea of the newborn (TTN) caused by delayed absorption of alveolar fluid. This condition may require oxygen therapy (Seidel *et al.* 1997) and admission to a special care baby unit.

Obstetric emergencies

There is a range of emergencies that can occur during labour that may have sequalae for the baby. These include antepartum haemorrhage, cord prolapse, shoulder dystocia and snapped cord and they are discussed in turn.

Antepartum haemorrhage

Antepartum haemorrhage (APH) can occur at any point during pregnancy or labour. The majority of APH occur as a result of either placenta praevia (in which the placenta is partly or totally lying over the cervical os) or placental abruption (the placenta separates from the uterine wall), which can be mild, moderate or severe (Lindsay 2004). An APH can be sudden and severe resulting in both maternal and neonatal compromise unless swift access to emergency care is achieved.

When the mother has had a series of small bleeds throughout pregnancy, but not so severe as to require emergency delivery, the placenta may have become chronically compromised and the baby may be growth restricted as a result. This is likely to have been identified antenatally if the woman presented for antenatal care.

Cord prolapse

This is an obstetric emergency that usually requires emergency caesarean section unless the woman's cervix is fully dilated and a swift instrumental birth is feasible. If the cord prolapses in front of the presenting part the blood supply to the fetus is occluded and the fetus can soon become asphyxiated. The attendant professional calls for help and endeavours to elevate the presenting part to reduce the pressure on the umbilical cord, by applying digital upwards pressure vaginally. The woman is manoeuvred into a knee–chest position and if there is time while waiting for theatre to become available a Foley catheter can be inserted into the bladder and 500 ml of saline infused. The management of cord prolapse is traumatic for all concerned as time is of the essence. It is likely that the woman will require the practitioner who examines her baby to reassure her that the baby has not been compromised.

Shoulder dystocia

Delay in delivering the fetal shoulders is a serious complication of the second stage of labour. Although the incidence of shoulder dystocia increases with fetal weight (Nesbitt *et al.* 1999; Mollberg *et al.* 2005), it is difficult to predict, and as such often comes as a shock to both the attendant and the woman. Following the birth of the head, the umbilical cord is compressed between the woman's pelvis and the baby's body. According to Baxley and Gobbo (2004) there are approximately seven minutes before a previously uncompromised baby becomes compromised. The most serious potential complication of shoulder dystocia is hypoxia, leading to death or permanent brain damage. The most common injuries following shoulder dystocia involve brachial plexus damage, resulting in one of three palsies: Erb's, Klumpke's or total brachial plexus (see Chapter 7). Occasionally the baby may sustain a fractured clavicle or humerus.

Snapped cord

If the cord snaps during the birth the attendant must ensure that, as soon as possible, a clamp is secured to the end attached to the baby first. Cases of snapped cord following water birth are particularly dangerous as they can go unnoticed for some time. They are most likely to result from applying undue traction to the cord after bringing the baby to the surface rapidly (Pairman *et al.* 2006). In very rare cases the baby may become anaemic and require a blood transfusion.

Resuscitation at birth

During your scrutiny of the mother's birth details it is important to note the condition of the baby at birth so that you may anticipate potential questions from the parents. All babies are given an Apgar score at birth, but this is not always conveyed to the parents. It is not appropriate that in your role as examiner of the healthy newborn infant you will be called upon to examine the severely birth-asphyxiated baby; such a baby would be carefully monitored in a neonatal unit. You will, however, examine babies who did require some form of resuscitation at birth, including administration of oxygen, oropharyngeal suction and intramuscular injection.

Resuscitation procedures are undertaken regularly by nurses, midwives and paediatricians. They are not, however, part of the daily repertoire of parents and can be alarming and confusing. The practitioner examining the baby can very simply clarify the confusion by saying, for example, 'I see from your notes that Hannah needed some oxygen when she was born because she did not want to breathe at first. She had some oxygen through a face mask and she became lovely and pink straight away. Her Apgar scores were fine (explaining what they are) and she came back to you. Is there anything you want to ask?' Such an explanation also reassures the parents that you know details about their daughter and are taking a thorough approach to her examination.

Injuries and abnormalities noticed at birth

It has already been seen that during the course of their birth some babies sustain an injury, such as a chignon, and these are discussed in more detail in Chapter 6. The purpose of mentioning them in the context of the first examination of the newborn is to remind the examiner to evaluate how the condition is progressing and whether it remains within the limits of normality. Recognising that an abnormality has been detected at birth, such as a birthmark, enables the practitioner to allocate a realistic length of time for the examination so that parents can ask extra questions that may have come to mind overnight. Parents may also need further information regarding subsequent care and, when possible, this should be reinforced through the availability of high-quality written information. National support groups for parents with children who have congenital abnormalities are detailed in Appendix 1.

Summary

Careful exploration of the birth records provides a wealth of valuable detail that will help with the examination of the newborn. It enables the examiner to provide personal, client-focused care and enhances the effectiveness of the procedure. As with all aspects of clinical practice, the practitioner must acknowledge when they are out of their depth and not attempt to deal with questions that they are not able to answer comprehensively.

The next chapter provides the reader with a systematic guide to undertaking the clinical examination of the healthy, term neonate and is the foundation from which normality can be confirmed and abnormality detected.

Self-test

1. What are the risks of prolonged pregnancy for the baby?
2. How are prolonged pregnancies managed where you work?
3. What is current practice regarding prelabour rupture of the membranes?
4. Why is it important to know if and why labour was induced in relation to examination of the newborn?
5. What is the normal fetal scalp blood pH?
6. What are the potential side-effects for the baby if the woman received pethidine during labour?
7. What might be the complications of a vaginal breech birth?
8. What is meconium aspiration syndrome?
9. What are the possible complications of an operative vaginal birth for the baby?
10. What factors should be considered when anticipating the effect of maternal analgesia on the neonate?

Activities

• Are women encouraged to have skin to skin contact with their baby following caesarean birth where you work? How is this practice monitored?
• Identify the policy for caring for women and babies when the membranes rupture before labour. Compare your unit's policy with that of a neighbouring unit and identify any differences.
• Consider what advice you would give to a mother who was leaving hospital and whose baby had a cephalhaematoma.

Resources

- The Baby Friendly Initiative. Information on breastfeeding. http://www.babyfriendly.org.uk/
- Cochrane database of systematic reviews related to pregnancy and childbirth. http://www.cochrane.org/reviews/en/topics/87_reviews.html
- Royal College of Midwives. Information to support high-quality care – practice guidance. http://www.rcm.org.uk/college/standards-and-practice/
- Royal College of Obstetrician and Gynaecologists guidelines. http://www.rcog.org.uk/womens-health/guidelines
- Royal College of Paediatrics and Child Health publications. http://www.rcpch.ac.uk/Publications/Publications-list-by-title
- The Information Centre. Information and statistics to support the delivery of high-quality care. http://www.ic.nhs.uk/

Chapter 6   Neonatal examination

- Introduction
- Step 1: preparation
- Step 2: observation
- Step 3: examination
- Step 4: explanation to the parent(s)
- Step 5: documentation
- Self-test
- Activities
- Resources

Introduction

This chapter is a step-by-step guide to the first examination of the newborn. It will take the practitioner systematically through the process and introduce the principles of neonatal examination. It will focus on the normal expected findings and also describe the abnormal findings that may be detected. It is through anticipation of the normal that deviations are detected, and this is the philosophy of the examination described in this chapter.

This chapter will describe five steps: preparation, observation, examination, explanation and documentation (Table 6.1). The management of abnormalities will be described in Chapter 7.

Step 1: preparation

The antenatal and labour records should be carefully scrutinised to identify any factors that might lead the practitioner to suspect potential concerns, as detailed in Chapters 3, 4 and 5 (for summary see Table 6.2). This preparation is also important so that the practitioner can approach the parents with an accurate history of what has happened to them, demonstrating that time and care have been taken to focus on this unique family unit.

Before the neonate is disturbed a great deal can be learned by listening to those who are caring for the mother and the baby and asking them if they have any concerns (Table 6.3). The parents should be encouraged to contribute information and ask any questions they may have during the examination.

TABLE 6.1 The five steps of neonatal examination

Step	Action	Description
1	Preparation	Read case notes (Table 6.2)
		Assess who is the most appropriate practitioner to undertake the examination
		Consider information from carers (Table 6.3)
		Gain verbal consent (see Chapter 8)
		Gather and clean equipment
		Wash and warm hands
2	Observation	Watch baby's behaviour
		Listen to the baby
		Listen to the parent(s)
3	Examination	Baby dressed
		Baby undressed
4	Explanation	Findings conveyed to mother
5	Documentation	Examination and action documented

TABLE 6.2 Points to look for in the maternal case notes

Problem/disorder type	Example(s)
Family history:	
Cardiac	Congenital heart disease and inherited conduction anomalies
Chromosome-related syndromes	Balanced translocation(s)
Developmental	Congenital deafness
Endocrine	Congenital adrenal hypo- or hyperplasia
Haematological	Haemoglobinopathies
Locomotor	Congenital dislocation of the hip
Metabolic	Galactosaemia
Neurodegenerative	Baton's disease
Neuromuscular	Spinomuscular dystrophy
Respiratory	Cystic fibrosis
Tumours	Retinoblastoma
Past medical history:	
Endocrine	Graves' disease, congenital hypothyroidism and diabetes
Haematological	Isoimmune thrombocytopenic purpura
Hypertension	Essential/pregnancy induced
Neuromuscular	Myasthenia gravis
Psychiatric	Postnatal depression
Medication	Teratogens, e.g. anticonvulsants, stilboestrol, thalidomide
Past obstetric history:	
Anomalies/disorders	Pre-term labour
Deaths	Sudden infant death
Infection	Cytomegalovirus
Social	Adoption/fostering
Present obstetric history:	
Expected date of delivery	Is the baby full term?
Conception	Donor
Habits	Alcohol, nicotine and drugs
Infection	Group B streptococcus, hepatitis B and C, herpes
Size	Abnormal/asymmetrical growth
Monitoring	Anomaly scans, glycosuria
Delivery details:	
Cardiotocograph anomalies	Decelerations
Delivery type and reason	Emergency section for fetal distress
Duration of membrane rupture	Prolonged rupture

TABLE 6.2 Continued

Problem/disorder type	Example(s)
Maternal medication	Opiates
Maternal well-being	Pyrexia
Baby:	
Condition of baby at birth	Apnoeic
Evidence of distress	Meconium passage *in utero*
Resuscitation details	Apgar scores, ventilatory support
Feeding	Breast/bottle
Vitamin K administered	Oral/intramuscular

It is important to anticipate and gather together the equipment that will be required during the examination and to ensure that it is clean (refer to local infection control guidelines) and in working order. The following is a list of equipment required to perform the neonatal examination:

- stethoscope;
- ophthalmoscope;
- spatula;
- tape measure;
- stadiometer (or equivalent);
- centile chart.

To have to leave the bedside to search for equipment might result in a previously contented baby becoming unsettled, hungry or in need of comfort, and the examination would then need to be postponed.

Informed consent

Very few parents will refuse to allow their baby to be examined; however, the practitioner should always ask the parent's consent before doing so (for further discussion regarding this issue see Chapter 8). Ideally, a parent should be present during the examination to allow exchange of information and advice as appropriate.

Step 2: observation

In addition, much can be learned about the neonate by looking and listening to him before disturbing him (Table 6.4). It is also wise to listen to the mother, who will already be the best judge of her baby's behaviour. Once all the information has been gathered from these sources the neonate can be disturbed.

TABLE **6.3** Points to listen out for from carers

	Observation(s)	Example(s)
Baby	Behaviour	Jittery, irritable, sleepy, etc.
	Feeding	Vomiting
	Monitoring	Pyrexia, colour, etc.
Mother	Behaviour generally	Tearful
	Behaviour towards baby	Caring, rough

TABLE **6.4** Observations before disturbing the neonate

Observation(s)	Example(s) of abnormalities
Colour	Cyanosis, pallor, plethora, jaundice
Cry	High pitched
Movement	Jittery, asymmetry
Posture	Hypotonia, Erb's palsy
Respiration	Recession, grunting, apnoea

Step 3: examination

Whoever performs the examination must be familiar with the art of clinical examination, which should always include the same four components:

1. looking (inspection);
2. feeling (palpation);
3. listening (auscultation);
4. tapping (percussion).

The first and third components are self-explanatory, but the second and fourth require some explanation of how they are performed, depending on which part of the body is being examined. Immediately before examining the baby the practitioner's hands should be washed and warmed.

Palpation is best performed with warm hands. It can give information about the firmness of underlying tissue (e.g. bony or cystic), the transmission of sound (e.g. murmurs or breath sounds), the size of and position of organs and the presence of masses. Palpation is performed differently depending on what information is being sought from what site and instructions will be given at the relevant points in the chapter.

Percussion can usually differentiate solid- or fluid-filled tissue from gas-filled tissue. It is performed by placing the middle finger of the left hand flat on the baby's body and gently tapping the middle phalanx with the middle finger of the right hand. This technique can be useful for examination of the chest (the percussion note is hyper-resonant in the presence of a pneumothorax) and abdomen.

The examination process

Examination of the baby is best performed with the examiner stood on the right-hand side of the bed with the baby lying with his head to the left of the practitioner.

One of the most difficult but important systems to examine is the cardiovascular system, for the baby must be calm and content. It is therefore prudent to examine the heart first. Initially, the neonate should be observed for cyanosis. His respiratory pattern should also be observed. The next steps are palpation and auscultation. Traditionally, these steps are performed with the neonate undressed, but beware as, although the neonate is born naked, he soon finds security in the closeness of clothing and removal of that clothing can result in a crying neonate. Under these circumstances, palpation and auscultation may not reveal any useful information about the heart. In the first instance it is worth attempting to palpate the chest and auscultate the heart with the neonate partially clothed. Successful examination of the heart sounds with the baby partially clothed does not preclude further examination of him when he is naked. However, if he then cries inconsolably when undressed, at least the heart sounds will have been heard and the presence of louder murmurs excluded.

Before undressing the neonate it also pays to concentrate next on the exposed parts of the baby (Table 6.5) and those areas that are best examined before the examiner puts her hands into a nappy full of meconium, i.e. eyes and mouth.

Once the exposed parts of the baby have been examined thoroughly the neonate may be undressed and the final stage of the examination begun (Table 6.6).

Scalp

The scalp is most commonly the presenting part at the birth. It is relatively easily traumatised and swelling with or without bruising is relatively common. A cranial meningocoele or encephalocoele may also produce a swelling. The scalp is also a common site for birthmarks or other skin abnormalities.

TABLE 6.5 Exposed parts of the baby

Part of body	Abnormalities to look out for
Scalp	Bruising/swelling
Head	Sutures and fontanelles
	Size
	Asymmetry/abnormal shape
Face	Characteristic facies, e.g. Down's syndrome
	Cleft lip
	Asymmetry
Mouth	Cleft lip
	Teeth
	Cysts
	Cleft palate
	Macroglossia
Ears	Skin creases, e.g. Beckwith–Wiedemann syndrome
	Deformity/absence
	Pre-auricular skin tags
Eyes	Absence
	Asymmetry
	Absent red reflexes
	Corneal opacities
	Coloboma
Neck	Extra skin folds
	Asymmetry
	Dimples
	Swelling
Hands and feet	Asymmetry/absence
	Skin creases
	Swelling
Arms and legs	Asymmetry/absence
Digits	Too few/too many
	Appearance of nails
	Appearance of digits
	Webbing

Head

Shape

The shape of the head can provide useful information, for example certain syndromes or sequences of abnormal development result in an abnormally

TABLE 6.6 Final part of the examination

Part of body/system	Abnormalities to look out for
Skin	Aplasia cutis
	Birthmarks
	Cuts or bruises
	Pigmentation
Chest	Shape
	Nipple position and number
Cardiovascular system	Heart position
	Heaves and thrills
	Heart sounds and murmurs (five spots)
	Peripheral pulses
Respiratory system	Respiratory effort
	Breath sounds
Abdomen	Distension/shape
	Organomegaly
	Tenderness
Umbilicus	Condition of cord
	Condition of surrounding skin
Male genitalia	Testes
	Shape and size of penis
	Position of meatus
	Urine stream
Female genitalia	Appearance
	Withdrawal bleeding
Anus	Patency
	Position
	Passage of meconium
Groin	Swelling
Hips	Stability
Spine	Deformity
	Overlying marks/defects
Central nervous system	Symmetry of reflexes
	Appropriateness of reflexes
	Ability to suck
	Tone
	Posture
Size	Weight
	Length
	Head circumference

shaped head, as does premature closure of certain sutures (craniosynostosis). A less worrying cause of asymmetry is a postural deformity acquired *in utero*; this will resolve with time.

Fontanelles and sutures (Figure 6.1)

Fontanelles are areas where at least three bony plates of the skull meet. They can be felt as soft spots on the head. The posterior fontanelle normally measures less than 0.5 cm at birth and closes shortly after it. The anterior fontanelle normally measures 1–5 cm in diameter at birth and does not close until 18 months of age. The anterior fontanelle at rest should neither bulge nor be sunken. It will bulge as the baby cries.

Sutures are the gaps between two bony plates of the skull. At birth, the sutures may be easily palpable, but the bone edges are not widely separated. Premature fusion of a suture may be palpable as a prominent edge. Likewise, over-riding sutures may be palpable as a prominent edge. This will resolve with time.

Size

The occipito-frontal head circumference is measured by placing a tape measure around the head to encircle the occiput, the parietal bones and the forehead (1 cm above the nasal bridge), that is, the largest circumference. This measurement should be repeated three times and the greatest measurement of the three is taken as being correct. There are centile charts available that take into account the baby's sex and gestation, but if these are not available the normal range for a term baby is 32–37 cm.

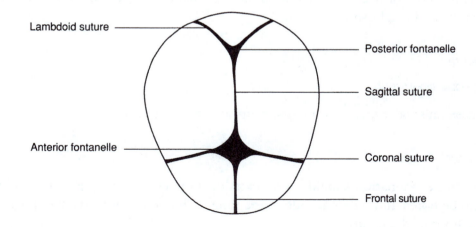

FIGURE 6.1 Fontanelles and sutures

Face

The face can be analysed as a whole or its components can be scrutinised individually (see below). The overall appearance of the face can be characteristic in certain syndromes, for example Down's syndrome, Crouzon's syndrome, etc. (see Chapter 7). Individual features in isolation do not necessarily indicate a syndrome, but in combination with other features they make a syndrome more likely. The practitioner should endeavour to see both parents before commenting on an unusual-looking face, as it may simply be familial.

It is also important to look at the symmetry of the face. Asymmetry may result from abnormalities of development of individual components, postural deformities or syndromes, for example hemihypertrophy, Goldenhar's syndrome (see Chapter 7).

Skin

The skin of the face should be uniform in colour, well perfused and free from swelling.

Nose

Babies are nasal breathers. The nose is often squashed *in utero* or during the birth, or it may not be completely patent. Occluding each nostril in turn will check for patency of the opposite nostril.

Lips

External abnormalities of the lips are usually obvious, but internal abnormalities are not necessarily so. Internal examination may require the use of a spatula and a light source.

Mouth

ALVEOLAR RIDGES (GUMS)

These must be inspected for cysts, clefts and neonatal teeth.

TONGUE

Careful examination should reveal cysts or dimples. The tongue size should also be noted and the underside of the tongue should be inspected along with the floor of the mouth.

This should be inspected carefully to exclude the presence of a cleft palate. It is not sufficient just to palpate the palate as clefts of the soft palate may be missed in this way.

Ears

These should be looked at for size, shape, position, abnormalities, for example skin creases, and surrounding anomalies, for example dimples and skin tags. Peculiarities should be discussed with the parents, for they may be familial.

Eyes

The practitioner should be familiar with the normal anatomy of the eye before examination (Figure 6.2). Check carefully to make sure there are two of them. Look at their size, their position (including distance of separation), the features around them (epicanthic folds, eyelids and eyebrows) and the slant of the palpebral fissures (Figure 6.3).

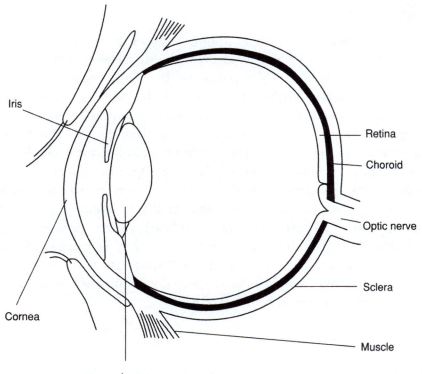

Iris

Retina

Choroid

Optic nerve

Sclera

Muscle

Cornea

Lens

FIGURE 6.2 Anatomy of the eye

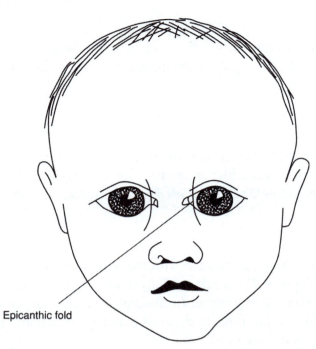

Epicanthic fold

FIGURE 6.3 Epicanthic folds

The sclera are normally white in colour. A yellow discoloration occurs with jaundice, the sclera may be blue in a baby with osteogenesis imperfecta (brittle bone disease) and it is relatively common for there to be haemorrhages following the birth. The iris of a baby is normally blue. It should be perfectly circular with a round opening (the pupil) in the centre. It usually appears to have fibres radiating out from the centre. The presence of white spots on the iris may be significant as they may associated with other conditions, for example Down's syndrome. The cornea and lens should be clear. Opacification may be secondary to congenital glaucoma, in which there is obstruction to the drainage of the eye, or a cataract (opacification of the lens). You should be able to elicit a red reflex by illuminating the eye with the ophthalmoscope set at +10 dioptres and held 15–20 cm from the eye. Failure to do so may be because of cataracts or a retinoblastoma (a tumour of the retina). Cataracts can be seen with the naked eye by shining a bright light tangentially. If there is any doubt, more detailed examination should be undertaken.

Neck

The neck may be shortened or webbed, or there may be restriction of the range of movement (congenital torticollis). The neck should have no abnormal swellings or dimples.

The clavicles should be examined for fractures, especially if there is any history of shoulder dystocia or any suggestion of an Erb's palsy.

Limbs

These should be of normal proportions, symmetrical and normally formed.

Hands and feet

The hands and feet are not normally puffy. They should be positioned in line with the limbs and be symmetrical to each other. There are usually multiple palmar creases and creases the entire length of the sole of the foot in the term baby.

Digits

Count the number of digits on each hand and foot. The digits should not be fused, shortened or abnormally shaped. The nails should be perfectly formed.

Chest

The chest should be symmetrical and there should be only two nipples, each situated just lateral to the mid-clavicular line, one on each side.

Cardiovascular system

When we refer to the cardiovascular system we do not refer solely to the heart, although for most parents this seems to be the most important part of that system. In our examination of the cardiovascular system the following should be considered:

- heart rate;
- heart rhythm;
- heart position;
- pulse volume;
- heart sounds (see p. 95 and Chapter 7).

In addition, the effort of the heart and its effect on other tissues, for example liver, oxygenation, etc., should be noted.

Congenital heart disease is said to have an incidence of 8 per 1000 live births (Haworth and Bull 1993). To be able to understand congenital heart disease, knowledge of the heart, its connections and the changes that occur following the birth is necessary.

From fetal to neonatal heart

In utero, the fetal heart and its connections allow the passage of most of the oxygen-rich blood from the placenta to the aorta via the right side of the heart, pulmonary artery and patent ductus arteriosus, with very little of it reaching the lungs (Figure 6.4).

After the birth, the placental supply of oxygen-rich blood is interrupted and only oxygen-poor blood from the body enters the right side of the heart. The lungs are inflated and the pressure required to perfuse the lungs falls. This results in the preferential perfusion of the lungs with this oxygen-poor blood. This blood becomes oxygenated in the lungs and is then returned to the left side of the heart, to be distributed to the body via the aorta. The increased oxygen content of the blood causes the ductus arteriosus to close and the relatively higher pressure on the left side of the heart causes the foramen ovale to close, resulting in the blood in the two sides of the heart being separated (Figure 6.5). These changes do not occur instantly – there is a gradual transition from one state to the other.

In the presence of a heart anomaly, the clinical findings and their time of onset are determined by the nature of the anomaly and the speed with which the changes (described above) occur. This means that not all heart anomalies will be detectable during the course of the neonatal examination.

Colour

Most babies are pink, although some babies exhibit acrocyanosis (cyanosis of the peripheries) without significance. Blue discoloration (cyanosis) occurs when blood becomes desaturated, that is, it carries less oxygen. Not all babies

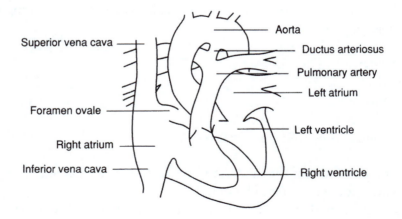

Figure 6.4 The fetal heart

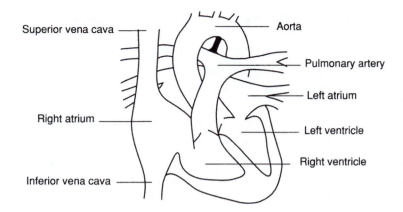

FIGURE 6.5 The neonatal heart and its connections

with congenital heart disease are cyanosed. When cyanosis is present, it can result from three different mechanisms:

1. low pulmonary blood flow;
2. transposition streaming;
3. complete intracardiac mixing.

Low pulmonary blood flow results from obstruction to blood leaving the right side of the heart (right outflow obstruction). Whilst the ductus arteriosus is patent, the lungs may be perfused by blood from the left side of the heart, but once the ductus closes pulmonary blood flow is reduced. The neonate then becomes cyanosed, but not usually breathless. In the absence of any septal defects left ventricular output may be reduced, but, if there is an accompanying septal defect, right-to-left shunting may occur and sustain left ventricular output. Examples of this include critical pulmonary stenosis, subvalvular obstruction as occurs in Fallot's tetralogy and, as an extreme case, pulmonary atresia (see Chapter 7).

Transposition streaming is a term used to describe the unfavourable streaming of desaturated blood from the vena cava into the aorta. Whilst the ductus arteriosus is patent, mixing of saturated with desaturated blood is possible. Once the ductus closes, unless there is an accompanying septal defect mixing cannot occur and the neonate develops two separate circulations. One circulation carries saturated blood from the lungs to the heart and back again and one carries desaturated blood from the body to the heart and back again. The neonate then becomes cyanosed, but breathlessness does not develop unless there is an accompanying septal defect.

Complete intracardiac mixing can occur at one of three levels:

1. *atrial*, e.g. unobstructed total anomalous pulmonary venous drainage;
2. *ventricular*, e.g. univentricular heart;
3. *great arteries*, e.g. truncus arteriosus.

The degree of cyanosis depends on the relative amounts of saturated (well oxygenated) and desaturated (poorly oxygenated) blood in the mixture and this in turn is dictated by the pulmonary blood flow (i.e. reduced pulmonary blood flow results in reduced saturated blood). Whether the neonate is breathless is also determined by the amount of pulmonary blood flow.

Heart rate and rhythm

The normal resting heart rate of a term neonate is approximately 90–140 beats per minute and the rhythm is normally regular. Minor variations in regularity can occur as a result of varying blood flow through the lungs with each breath.

Femoral pulses/pulse volume

Femoral pulses should be easily palpable in the groin of the neonate. Comparison of the femoral pulse volume with the brachial pulse volume (palpable in the antecubital fossa) may give further useful information, as may comparison of the right brachial pulse volume with the left brachial pulse volume. This part of the examination is best deferred until the groin is examined, but must not be forgotten.

Apical impulse

The apical impulse is normally palpable in the mid-clavicular line in the fifth intercostal space. It can give useful information as to the position of the heart.

Heaves/thrills

A heave is the term used to describe a diffuse impulse. A heave is best detected by placing the medial side of the hand on the chest wall in the region of the sternum (see Figure 6.6) and applying light pressure. The hand will be felt to lift very slightly with each cardiac impulse.

A thrill represents a murmur that is loud enough to be palpable. A thrill may feel like a cat purring or like a bluebottle trapped in the hand. Thrills are best appreciated during the expiratory phase of respiration, but for obvious reasons this is not always practical in a neonate.

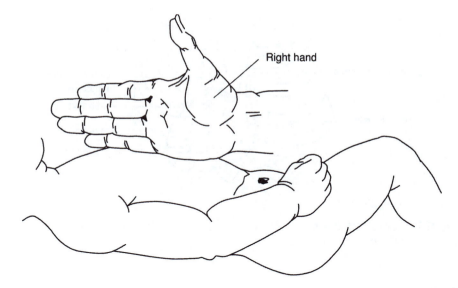

Right hand

FIGURE 6.6 Palpating the chest to detect a heave

Heart sounds

Normally only two heart sounds will be audible. Traditionally, the first heart sound is said to sound like 'lub' and the second to sound like 'dub'. The first heart sound (best heard at the apex) represents the closure of the mitral and tricuspid valves. The second heart sound (best heard at the second intercostal space) is actually split. The first component represents closure of the aortic valve and the second represents closure of the pulmonary valve. The split between these components normally becomes more evident during the inspiratory phase of respiration, but in a neonate, with a relatively rapid heart rate, the split is difficult to detect. Heart sounds are summarised in Table 6.7.

The human ear cannot normally detect the third and fourth heart sounds. The third heart sound represents ventricular filling that starts as soon as the mitral and tricuspid valves open, and the fourth heart sound represents ventricular filling that occurs in response to contraction of the atria.

TABLE 6.7 Audible heart sounds

Heart sound	Where	What
First	Apex	Closure of mitral and tricuspid valves
Second	Second intercostal space	Closure of aortic and pulmonary valves

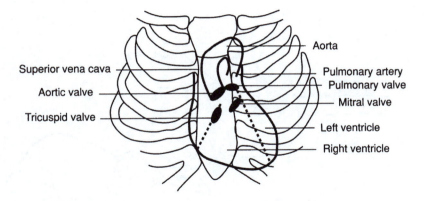

FIGURE 6.7 Position of the structures of the heart in relation to the surface markings of the chest

Murmurs

A murmur is an additional noise heard during the cardiac cycle. It is usually audible as a soft whooshing noise. To be able to interpret the relevance of a murmur, knowledge of the position of the structures of the heart in relation to the surface markings of the chest is needed (see Figure 6.7).

It is good practice to listen to at least five areas of the chest wall to exclude the presence of a heart murmur. These are:

1. the apex (mitral area);
2. the lower left sternal edge, at the fourth intercostal space (tricuspid area);
3. left of the sternum in the second intercostal space (pulmonary area);
4. right of the sternum in the second intercostal space (aortic area);
5. the midscapular area, posteriorly (coarctation area).

When listening for a murmur it is useful to palpate the brachial pulse simultaneously to determine whether a murmur is systolic or diastolic in timing and at what point in the cycle it occurs. If it occurs during the systolic phase of the cardiac cycle it occurs between the 'lub' and the 'dub' (see heart sounds above). A diastolic murmur is audible between the 'dub' and the next 'lub' of the heart sounds.

- An *ejection systolic murmur* starts just after the onset of systole and is maximal halfway through it.

- A *pansystolic murmur* extends throughout systole, starting at the same time as the first heart sound, and is accentuated slightly in mid-systole. It may extend slightly into diastole.
- An *early diastolic murmur* starts early on in diastole and is decrescendo.
- A *mid-diastolic murmur* starts later in diastole and is loudest in mid-diastole.
- A *presystolic murmur* occurs late in diastole.

The loudness of the murmur, which is graded from 1 to 6, should also be documented as follows:

- grade 1: just audible with the patient's breath held;
- grade 2: quiet;
- grade 3: moderately loud;
- grade 4: accompanied by a thrill;
- grade 5: very loud;
- grade 6: audible without a stethoscope and with the head away from the chest.

It is also not sufficient to assume that the murmur is audible only at that one position; it should also be documented whether the murmur radiates anywhere else.

Start by listening at the apex with the bell of the stethoscope. The diastolic murmur best heard at the apex with the bell of the stethoscope is that of mitral stenosis, which would be an unusual finding in a neonate. Next, listen over the lower left sternal edge (tricuspid area) with the diaphragm. Murmurs audible in this area with the diaphragm include the diastolic murmurs of aortic and pulmonary incompetence and tricuspid stenosis, and the systolic murmur of tricuspid incompetence. Next, listen over the second left intercostal space (pulmonary area) with the diaphragm. The murmur best heard in this area with the diaphragm is the systolic murmur of pulmonary stenosis. Next, listen over the second right intercostal space (aortic area) with the diaphragm to hear the systolic murmur of aortic stenosis. Finally, listen in the mid-scapular area with the diaphragm for the systolic murmur of a coarctation. The murmur of a valvular stenosis is often preceded by a click. This examination is summarised in Table 6.8.

Note that the absence of a heart murmur does not totally exclude a major cardiac anomaly. In an effort to increase the detection rate of cardiac abnormalities it is practice in some maternity units to combine physical examination of the cardiovascular system with:

- pulse oximetry in the air-breathing settled baby (Mahle *et al.* 2009);

TABLE 6.8 Examination of the heart

Where	How	What
Apex	Bell	Diastolic murmur: mitral stenosis
Lower left sternal edge	Diaphragm	Diastolic murmur: aortic and pulmonary incompetence
		Diastolic murmur: tricuspid stenosis
		Systolic murmur: tricuspid incompetence
		Pansystolic murmur: ventricular septal defect
Second left intercostal space	Diaphragm	Systolic murmur: pulmonary stenosis
Second right intercostal space	Diaphragm	Systolic murmur: aortic stenosis
		Systolic/pansystolic murmur: patent ductus arteriosus
Mid-scapular	Diaphragm	Systolic murmur: coarctation

Note: Absence of a heart murmur does not totally exclude a major cardiac anomaly.

- measurement of the post-ductal fractional oxygen saturation in one foot of all babies after the age of 2 hours and again before discharge (Richmond *et al.* 2002).

Liver size

The liver edge in a neonate is usually palpable anything up to 1 cm below the costal margin. It may be enlarged in the presence of heart failure.

Lung fields

When listening to the lungs there are usually only breath sounds audible, that is, the lung fields are usually clear. Fine crackles may be audible in the presence of heart failure.

Respiratory system

Colour

Not all babies with respiratory disease are cyanosed. Cyanosis can be a relatively late feature and is often preceded by pallor.

Respiratory effort

The neonate usually breathes without much effort. Respirations are usually quiet, chest movement is usually symmetrical and there is not normally any recession or use of accessory muscles of respiration.

Respiratory noises

A well baby normally breathes relatively quietly. Grunting is a term used to describe a noise that occurs when the neonate attempts to exhale against a partially closed glottis in an effort to avoid collapse of the alveoli. It may be present only when the neonate is disturbed or it may be present with every breath and be accompanied by other symptoms of respiratory disease.

Respiratory rate

Most neonates breathe around 40–60 breaths per minute. Their pattern of breathing is usually reasonably regular, but it is known for them sometimes to have periods of up to 10 seconds when they appear not to breathe. Rapid breathing (tachypnoea), erratic breathing or failure to breathe (apnoea) are all abnormal.

Air entry

When listening to the lungs there are usually only breath sounds audible, that is, the lung fields are usually clear. Air entry is usually symmetrical, but because of the relatively close proximity of the larger airways to the chest wall the breath sounds may sound bronchial in nature (like those heard over the throat or over a patch of pneumonia). This, combined with the relatively small surface area of the neonate's chest, makes it more difficult to differentiate between normal lung tissue and pneumonia in the neonate by auscultation alone. Crackles (crepitations) may indicate underlying infection, retained secretions, aspiration or heart failure. Wheeze (rhonchi) and stridor (a sound made during expiration) occur with airway obstruction.

Percussion note

The percussion note over the lungs is usually resonant. Pneumonia will give a dull percussion note and a pneumothorax will give a hyper-resonant note.

Abdomen

Colour

The abdomens of most babies are pink. Deviation from pink may indicate underlying pathology, for example a dusky colour may indicate an overly necrotic bowel, redness may indicate an overly inflamed bowel and a peri-umbilical flare may indicate local infection.

Shape

The abdomen is normally neither distended nor scaphoid (sunken). The shape can change depending on whether the baby has recently been fed, whether he is crying, whether the bladder is full or whether he has opened or is about to open his bowels. Extremes of shape can indicate underlying pathology, for example bowel obstruction, diaphragmatic hernia, etc.

Enlarged organs (organomegaly) and masses

In a baby the pelvis is relatively shallow and the diaphragm is not as deep. This means that some of the organs, which would not normally be palpable easily in an adult, become easily palpable if enlarged. The other two differences between a baby and an adult are:

1. babies are not generally obese – this makes palpation of organs and masses easier;
2. the spleen enlarges downwards rather than across and downwards (Figure 6.8).

Percussion of the abdomen may provide useful information; it can usually differentiate solid- or fluid-filled masses from gas-filled bowel.

Palpation is best performed by approaching from the right-hand side of the baby. The right hand is gently placed on the abdomen and superficial palpation is performed in all four corners of the abdomen and centrally. Once the baby is used to this, deeper palpation may be attempted. This is carried out by lying the index and middle fingers across the abdomen and gently but firmly stroking them up the abdominal wall or by gently pushing the tips of the same two fingers away from the rest of the hand.

*   *Palpation of the liver edge.* Start in the lower right quadrant and work slowly upwards towards the right subcostal (below the ribs) area. The procedure should be repeated centrally as the left lobe of the liver may be enlarged independently. A liver edge is normally palpable anything up to

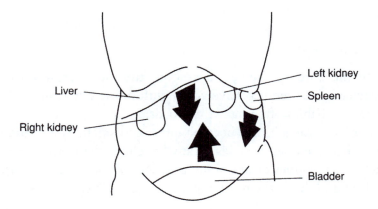

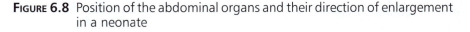

FIGURE 6.8 Position of the abdominal organs and their direction of enlargement in a neonate

1 cm below the costal margin. An edge palpable at greater than 1 cm may be abnormal.

- *Palpation of the spleen.* Start in the lower left quadrant and work slowly upwards. The spleen can be readily differentiated from the left kidney as it has a notch, which is relatively easily palpable, and it moves with respirations.
- *Palpation of the kidneys.* Place the left hand in the left loin and the fingers of the right hand on the front of the abdomen overlying the left hand. Gently push the left hand forward towards the right hand. Repeat this procedure on the right-hand side to palpate the right kidney. The right kidney may just be palpable, for it tends to lie lower down on the posterior abdominal because of the presence of the liver on the same side. The left is often impalpable.
- *Palpation of the bladder.* The bladder is often felt as a 'fullness' rising up from the pelvis.
- *Palpation of masses.* As with an intra-abdominal organ, any abdominal mass must be examined by means of inspection, palpation, percussion and even auscultation to have any idea of its origin. Knowledge of the stages of development of the contents of the abdomen is valuable as it may assist the identification of a mass, but it is beyond the scope of this book.

Tenderness

It is sometimes difficult to tell whether a baby has tenderness or not. Tenderness usually indicates underlying pathology, but it may be indicated only by a rigid abdomen, a crying baby or a baby who draws his knees up – all signs that may be found under other circumstances.

Umbilicus

Condition of umbilical cord

The size of the cord may give clues about the intrauterine growth of the baby – heavier babies tend to have cords with more Wharton's jelly whereas growth-retarded babies often have thin cords.

As the cord separates it may become moist and smell. Systematic review of the current evidence does not suggest any benefit to the routine use of topical agents such as antiseptics or antibiotic powders (Zupan *et al.* 2004). Keeping the cord clean and dry is the most appropriate care (NICE 2006).

Condition of surrounding skin

Around the time of separation, that is, between 5 and 15 days (Zupan *et al.* 2004), there is often a small degree of redness surrounding the attachment of the cord. This is usually unimportant, but if it begins to spread and extend up the abdominal wall it may indicate ascending infection that will require treatment.

Number of vessels in cord

When the cord is severed it is usually apparent that there are two arteries and one vein. There is an association of renal anomalies with cords with only one artery, but recent evidence suggests that this association is not sufficiently strong enough to justify further investigations (Deshpande *et al.* 2009).

Male genitalia

Scrotum

The scrotum may be relatively smooth or have a rugged appearance. It tends to have a mid-line ridge. A large scrotum may be the result of a hydrocoele. If this is the case it will transilluminate when a bright light is placed next to it in a darkened room. Occasionally, the scrotum develops as a bifid structure; the baby should be examined carefully to confirm that there are testes present in each half of it and that the rest of the genitalia are normal.

Pigmentation of the scrotum is common in babies born to parents who are not white, but it may be an early finding in congenital adrenal hyperplasia. Discoloration of the scrotum occurs with a neonatal torsion of the testis; the testicle is usually painful in this condition.

Testes

The scrotum is usually home to two testicles, which can be felt as two distinct entities, one in each side of the scrotum. Each testicle is approximately 1–1.5 cm in diameter, but may feel larger if there is an accompanying hydrocoele. In the absence of one testicle, the groin on the side of the absent testicle should be carefully palpated as the testicle may not have completed its descent from the posterior abdominal wall. It is also worthwhile palpating just below the groin as the testicle may have descended abnormally to that area. Absence of both testicles should alert the examiner to the fact that the baby's sex may be indeterminate. This will necessitate careful examination of the baby and further investigations.

Penis

The size of the penis at birth varies considerably, but if there are concerns about size there are centile charts for stretched penile length. There is little variation in the shape of the penis, but abnormalities can occur and include tethering of the penis to the scrotum, hooding of the foreskin, malpositioning of the meatus and incomplete development of the penis.

Female genitalia

Labia

As with the scrotum in the male baby, the appearance and colour of the labia are important things to note. Large labia may alert the practitioner to the fact that she is dealing with a baby of indeterminate sex and that there may be testes within them. They may also appear large in small-for-dates and preterm babies.

Pigmentation of the labia is common in babies born to parents who are not white, but it may be an early finding in congenital adrenal hyperplasia.

Vagina

The hymen may cover the vaginal orifice, and may be imperforate in some babies. Sometimes, vaginal skin tags are visible and may appear large in comparison with the labia. Shortly after birth, some babies suffer withdrawal bleeding and it is not uncommon for this to continue for several days.

Clitoris

The clitoris may seem quite large in small-for-dates and preterm babies, but its size must be assessed in comparison with its associated structures. If it is felt that it is inordinately large then the baby should be examined carefully to exclude an indeterminate sex.

Meatus

The position of the urinary meatus is a little more difficult to see in a female baby, but should be positioned between the clitoris and the vaginal orifice and the urinary stream should be good.

Anus

Patency

The patency of the anus is not always easy to assess. Even babies who have clearly been documented as having passed meconium within hours of birth have sometimes gone on to develop problems associated with patency because of a slightly malpositioned anus. It is important to take note of whether or not a baby has passed meconium. Delay in the passage of meconium beyond 24 hours should alert the examiner to the possibility of problems such as Hirschprung's disease, but it may also be delayed if the baby passed meconium *in utero*.

Position

The position of the anus in relation to the other perineal structures may alert the examiner to potential problems. An anteriorly placed anus may be associated with problems such as malformation of the rectum, constipation in later life, etc.

The examiner should also look carefully for evidence of leakage of meconium from sites other than the anus. Never assume that the meconium at the tip of the urinary meatus or covering the vaginal orifice is from the anus; it may be coming from a fistula (an abnormal connection with the rectum).

Groin

Perhaps one of the important things to determine here is whether or not the femoral pulses are palpable. The significance of this finding has been discussed in the cardiovascular section.

Swellings in the groin are not uncommon. They may be maldescended testes or hydrocoeles in the male baby, malpositioned ovaries in the female baby or herniae or vascular anomalies in either.

Hips

The hips should appear symmetrical; this includes the skin creases on the backs of the legs. They should also have a good range of movement, being fully abductable with no resistance to movement. Performing two manoeuvres should check the stability of the hips:

1. *Ortolani's manoeuvre*. If performed correctly this will detect a congenitally dislocated hip. The baby should be placed on his back on a firm flat surface. The legs are held with the hips and the knees flexed at right angles. The easiest way to do this is to hold the palm of the hand against the baby's shin, the thumb of the hand on the inside of baby's thigh and the middle finger overlying the greater trochanter of the femur. The hips are slowly abducted from the mid-line position through 90° while pushing forwards with the middle finger. A dislocated hip will clunk back into the acetabulum as this manoeuvre is performed. Failure to abduct the hips fully is suggestive of congenital dislocation, but not confirmatory. A click may be felt as a result of laxity of the ligaments of the hip or it may originate from the knee.

2. *Barlow's manoeuvre*. If performed correctly this will identify an easily dislocatable hip. With the legs held as for Ortolani's manoeuvre, pressure is applied to the front of the knee, forcing the femur to slide backwards. An unstable hip will dislocate out of the acetabulum. Performing Ortolani's manoeuvre can then relocate it.

If a dislocated or dislocatable hip is detected, the two manoeuvres should not be repeated, as there is a risk that the femoral head may suffer avascular necrosis. It should also be noted that it is practice in some maternity units to routinely scan the hips of breech babies and those with a strong family history of congenital dislocation of the hip as this has been shown to identify dislocation or dysplasia in asymptomatic babies (Lowry *et al.* 2005).

Spine

The spine is best examined by lying the baby face down with its abdomen and chest in the palm of one hand. The skin overlying the spine should be inspected, as an overlying abnormality of skin, for example a tuft of hair, swelling, pit or birthmark, may be an indication of an underlying abnormality.

Deformity can be easily seen, but it is also worthwhile feeling along the length of the spine to ensure that it runs a straight course.

Central nervous system

Behaviour

Take note of the everyday behaviour of the baby; a quiet baby may have a neurological problem, as may an irritable baby. Observe the baby's reaction to external stimuli; does he startle to loud noise, quieten to the spoken word, close his eyes in response to bright light, cry when undressed and cry when a feed is due?

Cry

In order to appreciate an abnormal cry the examiner has to be familiar with what a normal cry sounds like. The best way to do this is to spend time on a postnatal ward listening to babies cry.

Movement

Movement should be symmetrical inasmuch as both arms and legs should move equally and the muscles of the face should produce symmetrical expressions. Asymmetrical movement may indicate injury to nerve(s) (e.g. Erb's palsy), injury to bone (e.g. fracture of the clavicle), or neurological abnormality (e.g. Möebius sequence) (see Chapter 7).

Babies often appear to be jittery when they move. This probably represents an exaggerated response to movement. We forget that, as adults, we have had years to perfect our movements and that these movements have taken place in a free environment. Before birth babies are restricted by the confines of the uterus. They have never had to rely on the mechanisms that make our movements so precise. When they are born and those confines disappear they suddenly have freedom but not precision of movement, which results in them 'overshooting their mark' and appearing jittery. It is worth remembering that a baby can also be jittery because of low blood sugar (hypoglycaemia), infection, drug withdrawal, neurological problems and metabolic disorders.

Fits are not common in babies, but when they do occur they are often more subtle than those seen in adults and older children. They may be rhythmical jerking movements or they may be merely repetitive cycling or sucking movements, both of which can be subtle.

Posture and tone

When first born, a baby will often adopt the position he was in *in utero*. Soon after birth he begins to adopt a flexed/curled position. This change takes longer to achieve in the preterm baby, and there are charts available for assessment of posture with relation to gestational age (Ballard *et al.* 1991). A baby with reduced tone (hypotonia) may fail to flex, whereas a baby with increased tone (hypertonia) may adopt an extended position. Both posture and tone are controlled by the central nervous system, although neuromuscular problems will also affect both.

Hypotonia can be detected by supporting the baby by placing the hands one under each shoulder. A baby with normal tone will remain supported, but a baby with central hypotonia will 'slip' through the hands. Central hypotonia can be confirmed by lying the baby face down with its abdomen and chest in the palm of one of the practitioner's hands. A baby with normal tone will attempt to raise the head and the legs, but a baby with hypotonia will lie limply in the examiner's hand like a rag doll.

Hypertonia will often result in a rigid baby who does not exhibit head lag when pulled from the supine position to sitting. The baby's legs may be noted to 'scissor' or it may arch its back.

Reflexes

Perhaps the most important thing to take note of when assessing neonatal reflexes is whether or not they are symmetrical. The interpretation of neonatal reflexes must take place with the baby in a neutral (mid-line) position, as rotation of the head to one or other side during assessment can influence the findings.

The reflexes used to assess the neonate differ slightly from those used to assess older children and adults. In addition to the knee, ankle and biceps reflexes, which should be present, symmetrical and not exaggerated, there are also the Moro reflex, stepping reflex, rooting reflex, suck reflex and palmar and plantar grasp reflexes.

The *Moro reflex* is elicited by taking the baby in both hands, the head being supported by one hand and the buttocks by the other. With the baby's head in a mid-line position, the hand supporting it is quickly dropped to a position approximately 10 cm below its original supporting position and the head is caught by the hand in its new position. In response, the baby will throw out both arms and legs symmetrically.

The *stepping reflex* can be elicited by holding the baby under the shoulders with both hands. The baby's shin is placed in contact with the side of the cot and the baby will perform a stepping/climbing manoeuvre. This is repeated for the other leg.

The *rooting reflex* can be elicited by gently stroking the skin of the baby's cheek. He will turn the head towards the side that is being stimulated.

The *suck reflex* is elicited by placing the practitioner's clean little finger in the baby's mouth. The baby will suck on the finger as it would on a nipple or teat. Failure of the baby to suck may indicate underlying neurological damage, but before jumping to any such conclusion it is worth noting whether the baby has recently been fed and whether the baby is sleepy.

The *palmar grasp reflex* is elicited by placing the practioner's little finger into the palm of the baby. The baby's hand will grasp the practitioner's finger. Care should be taken not to touch the back of the hand at the same time as the finger is placed in contact with the palm as this can result in conflicting sensory information being presented to the neurones and an uninterpretable result being obtained.

The *plantar grasp reflex* is elicited by touching the sole of the baby's foot with the practitioner's little finger. The baby's toes will flex towards the practitioner's finger. Care should be taken not to touch the dorsum of the foot at the same time as the finger is placed in contact with the sole as this can result in conflicting information being relayed to the neurones and an uninterpretable result being obtained.

Assessment of intrauterine growth

Once this is complete, all that remains is to measure the baby's length and refer to the appropriate centile chart to check on size. Make sure you also plot the birth weight and occipito-frontal head circumference (see p. 87) at the same time.

Measurement of length can be a difficult procedure to perform correctly and requires the assistance of a second person and suitable equipment. Most hospitals have a stadiometer, which is a device for correctly measuring length; it is not sufficient to use a tape measure if an accurate assessment of length is required. The baby is placed on the stadiometer with his head firmly against the top end. The baby is then carefully stretched and the mobile bar is brought up to make contact with the flat of the baby's foot. The baby must be lying flat, with the head in contact with the top end of the stadiometer and the pelvis in a neutral position, that is, not tilted. The measurement is then read off the scale at the side of the stadiometer.

Use of centile charts is not difficult, but there is one peculiarity in their use. Although centile charts clearly have the weeks of gestation marked on their x-axis, a baby born at 36 weeks' gestation and above always has its birth measurements plotted as though it had been born at 40 weeks' gestation because it is deemed to be full term. Always make sure you have referred to the correct centile chart for the baby's sex and method of feeding and be aware that there are alternative centile charts for conditions such as Turner's syndrome and Down's syndrome, even though your hospital or practice may not routinely stock them.

Checklist

When the examination is complete, the examiner must make sure she has:

1. documented her findings (normal or abnormal);
2. informed the parents of any findings (normal or abnormal);
3. informed the paediatrician who is responsible for the care of the baby (abnormal);
4. informed the midwives caring for the baby and parent(s);
5. documented who was informed and when;
6. documented any action(s) taken;
7. provided the parents with the opportunity to ask further questions.

Step 4: explanation to the parent(s)

It is best practice to talk through the examination with the parent(s) while it is happening so that those questions that arise can be addressed in context. For example, as you are examining a baby's spine you can verbalize what you are expecting to find, 'I am feeling to see whether his backbone is in line and that there are no unusual lumps or dimples – and look, his spine is beautifully in line'. An examiner's careful concentration can easily be misinterpreted as concern, and therefore inadvertently raise anxiety levels in the parent(s). If you engage in conversation, it also makes it easier for concerns to be raised. If you conduct the examination in silence, parent(s) may be afraid to interrupt your concentration and therefore may not ask questions. It is also an opportunity to confirm the normality of features that may be alarming to the new mother or father, such as the shape of the baby's head after the birth or the appearance of the navel. Any abnormal findings must be conveyed to the parent(s) and this issue is discussed further in Chapter 7.

Step 5: documentation

The printed documentation of each trust will have a section within the baby notes that the practitioner must complete after the examination of the newborn. It usually comprises a checklist against which the practitioner can record her findings. Completing the records in view of the parent(s) provides another opportunity for reassuring the parents that all is well with the examination. Contemporaneous record keeping also helps avoid the potential errors of recall that may occur if records are completed some time after the event.

We have a professional duty to keep clear and accurate records of our observations and actions (General Medical Council 2006; Nursing and Midwifery Council 2004, 2008a, 2009) and this issue is discussed in further detail in Chapter 8 under the section 'Achieving and maintaining best practice'. Documentation should also include completion of the appropriate computer-based record and liaison forms, in line with trust policy.

The next chapter considers the identification of abnormal findings and how the practitioner examining the newborn infant should manage such discoveries.

Self-test

1. Why should Ortoloni's or Barlow's manoeuvres not be repeated when a positive result is obtained?
2. What is the normal range for a baby's respiration rate?
3. What is meant by the term 'craniosynostosis'?
4. How much of the liver should be palpable abdominally?
5. What is the normal range for a baby's head circumference?
6. List the five areas of the chest wall that should be listened to to exclude a heart murmur.
7. The 'lub' and the 'dub' heart sounds represent closure of which valves?
8. What might an anteriorly placed anus lead you to suspect?
9. What is the normal resting heart rate for a full-term infant at rest?
10. Describe how you would elicit the plantar grasp reflex.

Activities

- Identify five challenges to conducting the neonatal examination without interruptions. Now identify strategies to reduce the impact of such distractions in the hospital, the baby's home or the community clinic/children's centre. (*For example, your telephone or bleep may go off during the examination. A possible solution might be to negotiate a reciprocal arrangement with your colleagues to divert calls until the examination is complete and documented.*)
- Find out what information is available for new and prospective parents where you work on the examination of the newborn. In what form(s) is it available (e.g. written, web-based, DVD) and is it available in a range of languages relevant to the population? Who were the authors of the information and how often is it updated? How do you know that all parents receive such information?
- New parents often ask when a baby's eye colour might change. What would be your response?

Resources

- Examination of the newborn, Oslo University. Video clips and text available online. http://www.med.uio.no/learning-content/pediatrics-barnesykdommer/newborn/index.html
- NHS Antenatal and Newborn Screening Programmes. Newborn and 6- to 8-week Infant Physical Examination Digital Toolbox, prepared for the UK National Screening Committee. http://hearing.screening.nhs.uk/toolbox/index.php
- UK National Screening Committee policy database (neonatal). http://www.screening.nhs.uk/policies-newborn.
- NHS Newborn & Infant Physical Examination Programme (professionals). http://newbornphysical.screening.nhs.uk/professionals
- Continuing medical education resource. NetCE – Newborn Assessment Update. http://www.netce.com/coursecontent.php?courseid=502#PRENATALHISTORY

Chapter 7   Abnormal findings and congenital abnormalities

- Introduction
- Abnormal findings
- Specific abnormalities
- Specific syndromes
- Summary
- Self-test
- Activities
- Resources

Introduction

The aim of this chapter is to consider abnormalities that may be found during the first examination of the neonate and make suggestions regarding their appropriate management. It is important that the practitioner is able to recognise the significance of an abnormal finding and to differentiate between those that require:

- immediate medical attention;
- referral to a paediatrician or other specialist for follow-up;
- explanation or reassurance by the practitioner.

It is assumed that if an abnormality is discovered it will be discussed with a paediatrician, but the practitioner must be familiar with the local guidelines on investigation and management of individual conditions. The practitioner will also need to be familiar with normal laboratory values for the local hospital.

This chapter is divided into two major sections: abnormal findings and congenital abnormalities. The first section concentrates on individual abnormal findings and their relevance. The second section concentrates on the more common congenital abnormalities. Each section is arranged in a similar way to the previous chapter to enable the examiner to move between chapters and sections in the order that the baby is examined and in which abnormalities may be discovered. Whenever an abnormality is detected, the baby should be examined carefully to exclude other abnormalities.

Before embarking on the subject of abnormalities and how to deal with them there are several important things to remember when examining a baby in the neonatal period. This is an emotional period for both the mother and the father. Everyone expects that their baby will be perfect. To be told that a baby has or may have an abnormality can be devastating to some parents, especially the mother, who for the last 9 months has been the guardian of the baby and feels responsible for its growth and development.

The consequences of an abnormality can often be far-reaching, not only for the baby and parents but also for other members of the family. The child may have a reduced life span or may never fulfil his parents' expectations. His parents may have to devote time to unexpected hospital attendances and allow complete strangers access to their home and family. They may never be able to provide fully for their child's needs, relying on the support and expertise of outside agencies. Siblings may 'lose their place' in the family as the new addition puts increasing demands on time and energy. What was a solid family unit can sometimes be destroyed, resulting in the breakdown of that family.

Because of this, it is important to consider how, when and where parents should be told about an abnormal finding. Ideally, the news should be broken in the presence of support, for example with the partner present, in a private place and by someone who can explain in simple terms, without being patronising.

However one breaks 'bad news' to parents and family, in their eyes it will never be done perfectly, but it is up to the bearer of 'bad news' to try to attempt to do so. It is also important, once the news has been broken, to be available to answer questions and to have some understanding of the agencies that can offer support to the parents and family (see Appendix 1).

Abnormal findings

In Chapter 6 we have already suggested that a great deal of information can be obtained from the maternal notes. Indeed, we may well be alerted to the possibility of an abnormality just by checking the maternal notes (Table 6.2). Even if at first the maternal notes give us no clues as to the causes of a problem, it is always worth rechecking them. Some abnormal findings have common causes. To avoid repetition throughout the text, Tables 7.1 and 7.2 summarise the investigations and management that should be considered if certain common causes of abnormal findings are suspected.

Temperature instability

A temperature of up to 37.2°C is acceptable for a baby on a neonatal unit or a postnatal ward. A temperature of less than 36.5°C is considered to be hypothermic. Occasionally the environmental temperature can influence a baby's temperature, but other causes should be considered (see Table 7.1, p. 116).

Colour

Peripheral cyanosis

This is a blue discoloration of the skin of the hands and feet. It can occur when the baby is cold, but other causes should be considered (see Table 7.1, p. 116).

Central cyanosis

In central cyanosis, not only does the skin of the hands and feet and the remainder of the body have a blue discoloration, but also the lips, tongue and mucous membrane of the mouth. For causes see Table 7.1 (p. 116).

Anaemia reduces the oxygen-carrying capacity of blood and makes cyanosis more difficult to detect as it occurs only when the amount of desaturated haemoglobin is 5 g per 100 ml.

TABLE 7.1 Abnormal observations, possible causes and investigations to consider

Observations	Abnormality	Causes	Check maternal notes for evidence of	Possible causes and investigations to consider
Temperature	Instability	Intracranial haemorrhage Infection	Antenatal problems Difficult birth Difficult resuscitation Prolonged rupture of membranes Maternal infection	Consider investigating as for: infection, intracranial haemorrhage
Colour	Peripheral cyanosis	Cold peripheries Congenital heart disease Hypoxia	Difficult birth Difficult resuscitation	Check baby's temperature Consider investigating as for: congenital heart disease, hypoxia
	Central cyanosis	Congenital heart disease Infection Neuromuscular disease Respiratory disease	Prolonged rupture of membranes Maternal infection	Consider investigating as for: congenital heart disease, infection, neuromuscular disease, respiratory disease
	Pallor	Anaemia Hypoxia Infection	Fetal compromise Difficult birth Difficult resuscitation Prolonged rupture of membranes Maternal infection Maternal antibodies Blood group incompatibility Blood loss	Consider investigating as for: anaemia, hypoxia, infection

	Plethora	Pyrexia secondary to infection Polycythaemia	Prolonged rupture of membranes Maternal infection	Consider investigating as for: infection, polycythaemia
	Jaundice < 48 hours of age	Haemolysis Polycythaemia Infection (including hepatitis) Bruising Galactosaemia	Difficult birth Prolonged rupture of membranes Maternal infection Maternal antibodies Blood group incompatibility	Bilirubin Consider investigating as for: galactosaemia, haemolysis, infection (including congenital infection), polycythaemia
	Jaundice > 48 hours of age but > 10 days of age	Physiological Haemolysis Infection Bruising Galactosaemia	Difficult birth Prolonged rupture of membranes Maternal infection Maternal antibodies Blood group incompatibility	Bilirubin If there is any reason to suspect anything other than physiological jaundice proceed to investigate as for jaundice < 48 hours of age
Behaviour	Abnormal cry	Hypoxia Raised intracranial pressure Infection Neurodevelopmental abnormalities Certain syndromes	Antenatal problems Fetal compromise Difficult birth Difficult resuscitation Prolonged rupture of membranes Maternal infection	Consider investigating as for: hypoxia, infection, neurodevelopmental abnormalities, raised intracranial pressure, syndrome
	Abnormal posture	Hypoxia Raised intracranial pressure Intracranial haemorrhage Infection Neurodevelopmental abnormalities Nerve or bone trauma Hyperbilirubinaemia causing kernicterus	Antenatal problems Fetal compromise Difficult birth Difficult resuscitation Prolonged rupture of membranes Maternal infection	Bilirubin Consider investigating as for: hypoxia, infection, intracranial haemorrhage, neurodevelopmental abnormalities, raised intracranial pressure

TABLE 7.1 Continued

Observations	Abnormality	Causes	Check maternal notes for evidence of	Action/investigation
	Irritable	Hypoxia Raised intracranial pressure Intracranial haemorrhage Infection Neurodevelopmental abnormalities Withdrawal from maternal medication or maternal drugs Pain, e.g. from trauma	Fetal compromise Difficult birth Difficult resuscitation Maternal medication Maternal drug abuse Prolonged rupture of membranes Maternal infection	Urine toxicology screen on baby and mother Consider investigating as for: hypoxia, infection, intracranial haemorrhage, neurodevelopmental abnormalities, raised intracranial pressure
	Sleepy	Hypoglycaemia Hypermagnesaemia Infection Hyperbilirubinaemia Maternal medication Maternal drug abuse	Maternal medication Maternal drug abuse Maternal glucose intolerance Maternal infection Prolonged rupture of membranes	Blood glucose Bilirubin Magnesium Urine toxicology screen on baby and mother Consider investigating as for: infection
Feeding	Vomiting	Hypoxia Raised intracranial pressure Infection Maternal medication or maternal drug abuse Gastrointestinal abnormalities Congenital adrenal hyperplasia Galactosaemia	Fetal compromise Difficult birth Difficult resuscitation Maternal medication Maternal drug abuse Prolonged rupture of membranes Maternal infection	Urine toxicology screen on baby and mother Blood urea and electrolytes 17-hydroxyprogesterone (at > 48 hours of age) Abdominal radiography with or without contrast Abdominal ultrasound Consider investigating as for: galactosaemia, hypoxia, infection, raised intracranial pressure

	Inability to suck or feed	Prematurity Cleft lip or palate Jaundice Neurodevelopmental abnormalities	Prematurity Fetal compromise Difficult birth Difficult resuscitation	Bilirubin Refer to cleft lip and palate team if either is present Consider referring to speech therapist Consider investigating as for: neurodevelopmental abnormalities
Movement	Asymmetry	Ischaemia Haemorrhage Neurodevelopmental abnormalities Nerve or bone injury	Fetal compromise Difficult birth Difficult resuscitation	Consider investigating as for: bone injury, ischaemia, neurodevelopmental abnormalities
	Fits	Hypoxia Raised intracranial pressure Haemorrhage Infection Neurodevelopmental abnormalities Hypocalcaemia Hypoglycaemia Maternal medication or maternal drug abuse	Fetal compromise Difficult birth Difficult resuscitation Maternal medication Maternal drug abuse Prolonged rupture of membranes Maternal infection Glucose intolerance	Calcium Glucose Urine toxicology screen on baby and mother Consider investigating as for: hypoxia, infection, intracranial haemorrhage, neurodevelopmental abnormalities, raised intracranial pressure

TABLE 7.1 Continued

Observations	Abnormality	Causes	Check maternal notes for evidence of	Action/investigation
	Jittery	Hypoxia Haemorrhage Infection Neurodevelopmental abnormalities Hypocalcaemia Hypoglycaemia Maternal medication or maternal drug abuse Exaggerated normal response	Fetal compromise Difficult birth Difficult resuscitation Maternal medication Maternal drug abuse Prolonged rupture of membranes Maternal infection Glucose intolerance	Calcium Glucose Urine toxicology screen on baby and mother Consider investigating as for: hypoxia, infection, intracranial haemorrhage, neurodevelopmental abnormalities, raised intracranial pressure
Chest	Asymmetry	Abnormalities of external structures of the chest pneumothorax Diaphragmatic hernia		Consider investigating as for: respiratory disease
	Fast or slow heart rate		Maternal medication Maternal drug abuse Maternal disease, e.g. systemic lupus erythematosus (SLE) or Graves' disease	ECG Thyroid function tests Urine toxicology screen on baby and mother Consider discussing with a cardiologist if heart rate > 240 beats per minute or there is heart block; treating the baby for thyrotoxicosis if present

Finding	Cause	Risk factors	Action
Reduced femoral pulse volume or absent femoral pulses	Left ventricular outflow obstruction Infection	Prolonged rupture of membranes Maternal infection	Consider investigating as for: infection, congenital heart disease
Displaced apical impulse	Dextrocardia (heart on the opposite side to normal) Cardiomegaly (enlarged heart) Pneumothorax (air in the thoracic cavity)		Locate the apical impulse by palpation Chest radiography Consider referring to cardiologist for cardiomegaly or dextrocardia Consider investigating as for: respiratory disease
Heave/thrill palpable	Congenital heart disease		Consider investigating as for: congenital heart disease
Abnormal heart sounds	Congenital heart disease		Consider investigating as for: congenital heart disease
Murmur	Congenital heart disease Anaemia	Maternal antibodies Blood group incompatibility Blood loss	Consider investigating as for: congenital heart disease, anaemia
Recession	Choanal atresia Pneumothorax Infection	Prolonged rupture of membranes Maternal infection	Exclude choanal atresia Consider investigating as for: respiratory disease, infection

TABLE 7.1 Continued

Observations	Abnormality	Causes	Check maternal notes for evidence of	Action/investigation
	Grunting	Infection Hypoglycaemia Respiratory distress syndrome Diaphragmatic hernia Pneumothorax Hypoplastic lungs Congenital heart disease	Prematurity Glucose intolerance Prolonged rupture of membranes Maternal infection	Blood sugar Consider investigating as for: infection, respiratory disease, congenital heart disease
	Tachypnoea	Congenital heart disease Respiratory disease, e.g. respiratory distress syndrome Respiratory abnormality, e.g. diaphragmatic hernia, pneumothorax Metabolic disease Infection	Prematurity Prolonged rupture of membranes Maternal infection	Consider investigating as for: infection, respiratory disease, congenital heart disease, metabolic disease
	Irregular/ gasping respirations	Hypoxia Congenital heart disease Respiratory disease Respiratory abnormality Maternal opiates Infection Immaturity of the respiratory centre Metabolic disease Neurological disease	Prematurity Fetal compromise Difficult birth Difficult resuscitation Maternal medication Maternal drug abuse Prolonged rupture of membranes Maternal infection	Urine toxicology screen on baby and mother Consider investigating as for: hypoxia, infection, respiratory disease, congenital heart disease, metabolic disease, neuromuscular disease

	Sign	Causes	Contributory factors	Investigation
	Apnoea	Maternal opiates Infection Immaturity of the respiratory centre Choanal atresia Neurological disease	Prematurity Maternal medication Maternal drug abuse Prolonged rupture of membranes Maternal infection	Exclude choanal atresia Urine toxicology screen on baby and mother Consider investigating as for: infection, neuromuscular disease
	Unequal air entry or added sounds	Infection Pneumothorax Heart failure Upper airway obstruction	Prolonged rupture of membranes Maternal infection	Consider investigating as for: infection, respiratory disease, congenital heart disease
Abdomen	Discoloration	Infection Bowel obstruction Ischaemic/necrotic bowel	Prolonged rupture of membranes Maternal infection Difficult birth	Abdominal radiography Consider investigating as for: infection
	Hepatomegaly	Congenital heart disease Heart failure Congenital infection Metabolic conditions Intrahepatic haemorrhage Vascular anomalies Tumours		Glucose Liver function tests Clotting screen (liver ultrasound) Consider investigating as for: congenital heart disease, metabolic disease, congenital infection
	Splenomegaly	Haemolysis Infection Congenital infection Trauma	Difficult birth Prolonged rupture of membranes Maternal infection Maternal antibodies Blood group incompatibility	Bilirubin (spleen ultrasound) Consider investigating as for: haemolysis, infection, congenital infection

TABLE 7.1 Continued

Observations	Abnormality	Causes	Check maternal notes for evidence of	Action/investigation
Genitalia	Pigmentation	Ethnic origin Congenital adrenal hyperplasia	Blood electrolyte levels	Consider checking: 17-hydroxyprogesterone levels at 48 hours of age
Central nervous system	Reduced tone or increased tone	Hypoxia Raised intracranial pressure Intracranial haemorrhage Infection Neurodevelopmental abnormalities	Fetal compromise Difficult birth Difficult resuscitation Maternal medication Maternal drug abuse Prolonged rupture of membranes Maternal infection	Urine toxicology screen on baby and mother Consider investigating as for: hypoxia, infection, intracranial haemorrhage, neurodevelopmental abnormalities, raised intracranial pressure, syndrome
	Asymmetrical reflexes	Hypoxia Raised intracranial pressure Intracranial haemorrhage Neurodevelopmental abnormalities Bone or nerve injury	Fetal compromise Difficult birth Difficult resuscitation	Urine toxicology screen on baby and mother Consider investigating as for: hypoxia, intracranial haemorrhage, neurodevelopmental abnormalities, raised intracranial pressure, bone trauma

Pallor

The skin is pale in colour. For causes see Table 7.1 (p. 116).

Plethora

The skin is red or deep pink in colour. For causes see Table 7.1 (p. 117).

Jaundice

This is a yellow discoloration of the skin and sclera of the eyes. It occurs when the level of circulating bilirubin becomes elevated. This commonly occurs in the newborn baby about 3 days after delivery as a result of increased red cell breakdown and immaturity of the liver. Jaundice occurring earlier than this, and especially within 24 hours of delivery, usually requires investigation as does jaundice occurring after 10 days of age. It is also worth considering the possibility of abnormal causes of jaundice in a baby who develops it within the period 3–10 days of age. For causes see Table 7.1 (p. 117).

Behaviour

Abnormal cry

To appreciate an abnormal cry the examiner has to be familiar with what a normal cry sounds like. The best way to do this is to spend time on a postnatal ward listening to the crying of babies. An example of an abnormal cry is a high-pitched cry. For causes see Table 7.1 (p. 117).

Abnormal posture

When a baby is first born it usually adopts the posture it had *in utero*, for example an extended breech baby will attempt to lie with its hips flexed and its feet almost up by its ears. Gradually the baby adopts a flexed posture with elbows, knees and hips flexed. For causes of abnormal posture see Table 7.1 (p. 117).

Irritability

Most babies cry at some time, but they are generally consolable by picking them up and comforting them, changing their nappy or feeding them. A baby who cannot be consoled may have an underlying reason for this (see Table 7.1, p. 118).

TABLE 7.2 Observed conditions with suggested investigations in management

Causes	Check maternal notes for evidence of	Investigation	Possible finding	Management
Anaemia	Blood loss Blood group incompatibility Maternal antibodies	Haemoglobin Direct Coombs test Blood group (mother and baby) Maternal Kleihauer test	Low haemoglobin Positive result Incompatability Positive with feto-maternal bleed	Correction of anaemia Monitor bilirubin and haemoglobin Supplemental folic acid Check bilirubin
Bone trauma		Radiograph	Fracture/dislocation	Discussion with orthopaedic surgeon
Congenital heart disease	ECG	Chest radiograph Hyperoxia test Four-limb blood pressure Echocardiogram Oxygen saturation measurement	Depends on cardiac lesion	Depends on cardiac lesion, e.g. prostaglandins for duct-dependent lesions
Congenital infection	Maternal infection	Toxoplasma titres Rubella titres Cytomegalovirus (urine culture and throat swab) Hepatitis B and C Platelet count Liver function tests	Result not immediately available May be < $150 \times 10^9/l$ May be deranged	

126

Condition	Causes	Investigation	Result	Management
Galactosaemia		Urine-reducing substances	Positive	Lactose-free milk
		Red blood cell galactose-1-phosphate-uridyl-transferase level	Reduced	
		Liver function tests	May be deranged	
Haemolysis	Blood group incompatibility	Bilirubin	Raised	Phototherapy
	Maternal antibodies	Haemoglobin	Low	Check bilirubin
	Maternal infection	Blood group (mother and baby)	Incompatible	
		Direct antiglobulin test	Positive	
		Blood film	Abnormal-shaped red cells	
		Red cell enzymes, e.g. glucose-6-phosphate dehydrogenase level	Low levels	
		Consider investigating as for infection		
Hypoxia	Fetal compromise	Arterial blood gas	Hypoxia	Oxygen
	Difficult birth		Metabolic acidosis (base excess $\geq$ 10 mmol/l)	Ventilatory support
	Difficult resuscitation			Correction of acidosis

TABLE 7.2 Continued

Causes	Check maternal notes for evidence of	Investigation	Possible finding	Management
Infection	Prolonged rupture of membranes Maternal infection	White blood cell count	Raised (refer to laboratory values)	Antibiotics
		Platelet count	$< 150 \times 10^9$/l	
		Erythrocyte sedimentation rate	> 10 mm/h	
		C-reactive protein	> 10 g/l	
		Blood culture	Result not immediately available	
		Surface swabs		
		Urine culture (lumbar puncture)		
Intracranial haemorrhage	Antenatal problems Difficult birth Difficult resuscitation	Cranial ultrasound	May be normal immediately after the haemorrhage	
Ischaemia	Antenatal problems Difficult resuscitation Difficult birth	Cranial ultrasound (CT scan, MRI scan)		

Condition	Investigation	Result	Management
Metabolic disease	Blood glucose	Low	Consider checking insulin and cortisol levels Treat hypoglycaemia
	Arterial blood gas	May show metabolic acidosis (base excess ≥ 10)	Correction of acidosis
	Urine-reducing substance	May be positive	Identify reducing substance and treat if necessary
	Urine amino and organic acids	May indicate disorder of amino/organic acid pathways	Discuss with consultant with interest in metabolic disorders
	Ammonia	Raised in urea cycle defects	
Neurodevelopmental abnormalities	Cranial ultrasound (CT scan, MRI scan)		Discussion and/or referral to a neurologist or neurosurgeon may be necessary
Neuromuscular disease			Discussion and/or referral to a neurologist may be necessary
Polycythaemia	Full blood count	Raised haemoglobin	Dilutional exchange transfusion Haematocrit > 60%
	Glucose	Hypoglycaemia	Supplemental glucose
	Bilirubin	Raised	Phototherapy

TABLE 7.2 Continued

Causes	Check maternal notes for evidence of	Investigation	Possible finding	Management
Raised intra-cranial pressure		Cranial ultrasound (CT scan, MRI scan)		Discussion and/or referral to a neurosurgeon may be necessary
Respiratory disease		Transillumination of the chest	Chest transilluminates with pneumothorax	Thoracocentesis (temporary drainage) Chest drain insertion
		Chest radiograph	May show pneumonia; respiratory distress syndrome; pneumothorax	Respiratory support, e.g. oxygen, ventilation; antibiotics for pneumonia; drainage of a symptomatic pneumothorax
		Arterial blood gas	Low PaO_2, raised $PaCO_2$, pH < 7.25	
Syndrome	Family history	Chromosome analysis	May be normal	Genetic advice

Sleepy

The majority of babies sleep for most of the day, but they do tend to wake for feeds. Excessive sleepiness is abnormal. For causes see Table 7.1 (p. 118).

Inability to feed or suck

This may alert the practitioner to examine for prematurity (assess gestational age) and exclude physical anomalies such as cleft palate. Jaundice may also render the baby reluctant to feed, or there may be a neurodevelopmental abnormality requiring further investigation (see Table 7.1, p. 119).

Vomiting

Most babies will vomit at some time. Frequent large vomits are abnormal and a cause should be sought (see Table 7.1, p. 119).

Bile-stained vomit (green or yellow) is abnormal and is more likely to indicate obstruction. Blood-stained vomit may be the result of ingestion of maternal blood, trauma or a coagulation problem (excluded by checking clotting and platelet count). Babies frequently bring up small quantities of milk with wind (a possit). This is of no significance.

Movement

Asymmetry

Babies should be capable of moving both sides of their body to the same degree – not necessarily at the same time! If movement appears to be asymmetrical there may be an underlying cause (see Table 7.1, p. 119).

Fits

At some point in time most babies will exhibit jerking movements. Determining which of these movements are normal and which are abnormal can be difficult. Jerking movements of the limbs that settle when the limb is held are usually not significant, but those that do not settle may well represent a fit. Other movements that may represent a fit include 'cycling' movements of the arms and legs. Sometimes the only evidence of a fit is a dusky (slightly cyanosed) baby, resulting from a brief cessation of breathing (an apnoea attack) caused by the fit. For causes of fits see Table 7.1 (p. 119).

Fits should be referred to a paediatrician. Those that are prolonged or are causing neonatal compromise (apnoea, cyanosis and distress) may require treatment.

Jittery

A 'jitter' is a rhythmical movement of the arms and legs that settles when the limbs are steadied. It can be a normal finding (an exaggerated normal response), but it may have an underlying cause (see Table 7.1, p. 120).

Scalp

Bruises/swelling

Bruising and swelling are common responses to trauma. Both will resolve with time. Bruising may contribute to the development of jaundice.

Caput succedaneum (Figure 7.1)

This is subcutaneous oedema resulting from prolonged labour. It may present with or without bruising, and crosses suture lines. This is a benign finding that will resolve fairly quickly.

Cephalhaematoma (Figure 7.2)

A cephalhaematoma is when trauma causes subperiosteal haemorrhage confined to the skull bone(s). Swelling is contained within the suture lines but may

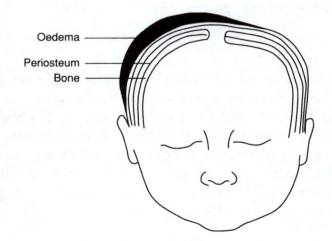

FIGURE 7.1 Caput succedaneum

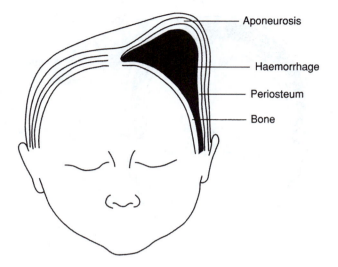

FIGURE 7.2 Cephalhaematoma

be unilateral or bilateral. This is a benign finding that will gradually resolve and may contribute to the development of jaundice. The swelling should not increase in size significantly after the birth.

Subaponeurotic haemorrhage (Figure 7.3)

Trauma to the scalp can cause a subaponeurotic haemorrhage not confined to a bone. The haemorrhage may be sufficient to necessitate resuscitation with intravenous fluids. Haemoglobin estimation may give some estimate of volume of blood loss, although the result may be misleading. Transfusion is likely to be necessary. A clotting screen may be abnormal because of the consumption of clotting factors, and treatment with cryoprecipitate, platelets and vitamin K may be necessary.

Meningocoeles and encephalocoeles

These are usually found at the occiput in the mid-line. They are usually associated with a bony defect of the cranium. A meningocoele contains meninges, that is, the layers covering the spinal column, but not any neural tissue. An encephalocoele contains meninges and neural tissue. They may also be associated with an abnormal neurological examination. A cranial ultrasound will confirm the diagnosis, although a skull radiograph and a cranial computerised tomography (CT) or magnetic resonance imaging (MRI) scan may also be required. Discussion and/or referral to a neurosurgeon will be necessary.

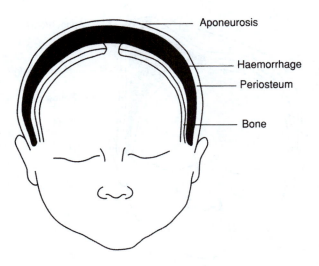

- Aponeurosis
- Haemorrhage
- Periosteum
- Bone

FIGURE 7.3 Subaponeurotic haemorrhage

Face

Asymmetry

Asymmetry may be the result of the baby lying awkwardly *in utero*, but it can occur with syndromes such as Goldenhar's syndrome (see p. 179), and it can occur in association with hemihypertrophy (enlargement of one side of the body). Hemihypertrophy may also be associated with nephroblastoma (a renal tumour).

In the case of a postural deformity, the only action necessary is to explain to the parents that this is usually a benign finding that will resolve fairly quickly. If there is associated hemihypertrophy a renal ultrasound scan should be arranged. It may be necessary to enlist the services of a geneticist to identify a syndrome if one is suspected. Severe facial abnormalities may benefit from referral to a craniofacial surgical team.

Small jaw

This may be familial or it may occur as part of a syndrome, for example Pierre Robin's syndrome (see p. 177). The first thing to do is to take a close look at the parents. If you suspect that Pierre Robin's syndrome is likely, be sure to look for an associated cleft palate.

Dysmorphic facies

These may be familial, so always look at the parents. They can also occur in certain syndromes, for example Goldenhar's, Down's and Turner's syndromes (see pp. 175–80), and in association with metabolic conditions, for example mucopolysaccharidoses and congenital hypothyroidism.

If you suspect a syndrome look for other features associated with the syndrome. Chromosome analysis may assist in confirmation or identification of a syndrome. It may be necessary to enlist the services of a geneticist to identify a syndrome if one is suspected.

Birthmarks (see Skin, pp. 143–8)

There are many types of birthmarks, but those occurring most commonly in the neonatal period are described below.

Salmon patch naevus (Plate 4)

This flat, ill-defined pink or red birthmark usually fades within the first year. Salmon patch naevus does not require intervention.

Port wine stain (Plate 5)

Port wine stain in the distribution of the first branch of the trigeminal (third cranial) nerve may be associated with vascular malformation of the meninges and cerebral cortex on the same side. Radiological investigation, for example cerebral ultrasound, CT scan or MRI scan, will help to exclude such involvement and should be considered. Referral to a dermatologist for cosmetic treatment should also be considered. Port wine stains around the eye may be associated with glaucoma and so an ophthalmological opinion should be sought to exclude this.

Strawberry haemangioma (Plate 6)

A haemangioma is a benign, vascular growth from the skin. This firm red lesion may need to be referred to a dermatologist if it involves the eyelid or has a potential to obstruct vision in the early years. A strawberry haemangioma will show a rapid growth spurt and then will resolve over the course of the next 2 years.

Cavernous haemangioma (Plate 7)

This red-blue haemangioma encloses large blood-filled vessels and should be referred to a dermatologist for assessment and ongoing monitoring. After initial proliferation, haemangioma usually involute spontaneously, although some require laser or steroid therapy.

Nose

Obstruction

Failure of the nasal passages to become patent may cause obstruction (unilateral or bilateral choanal atresia), as may deviation of the nasal septum. Bilateral choanal atresia requires urgent treatment, which consists of establishing a patent airway and urgent referral to an ear, nose and throat (ENT) surgeon. Unilateral choanal atresia also requires referral to an ENT surgeon, but the urgency is not quite as great as with a bilateral atresia. A deviated nasal septum may require referral to an ENT surgeon.

Mouth

Neonatal teeth

Teeth present at or shortly after birth are not common but should be referred to the orthodontic team, as they may be quite loose and can be inhaled if not removed electively.

Cleft lip

This condition is sometimes detected in the antenatal period. In such cases the baby should be automatically referred to the local cleft lip and palate team (plastic surgeon, ENT surgeon, audiologist, orthodontic surgeon and speech therapist) before the birth. Those babies who did not have the condition detected antenatally should be referred to the cleft lip and palate team as soon as possible after delivery and examined by a paediatrician. It is worth noting that women whose babies did not have the condition detected antenatally may feel betrayed and confused and require a lot of support. Practitioners should be familiar with local policies and resources regarding:

- the timing of surgical closure of the cleft;
- equipment to help with feeding difficulties;
- photographs showing babies before and after surgical repair;
- local and national support groups (see Appendix 1).

Cleft lip may be familial but it may occur spontaneously or as a result of chromosomal abnormalities (e.g. Patau's syndrome; see p. 178), or maternal medication (e.g. phenytoin). Look carefully for an associated cleft palate and for other features that might suggest a syndrome.

Cleft palate

This may occur in isolation or in association with cleft lip. It may be familial or may occur spontaneously or as a result of a chromosomal abnormality (e.g. Patau's syndrome; see p. 178), or maternal medication (e.g. phenytoin).

As with cleft lip, cleft palate may be diagnosed antenatally and should be referred to the cleft lip and palate team as soon as it is diagnosed.

Cysts

RANULAE

Ranulae are mucus retention cysts and appear as blue lumps beneath the anterior part of the tongue. They may be large enough to displace the tongue posteriorly and interfere with respirations. In the event of this happening they can be aspirated, but they are usually left alone if they do not interfere with feeding or breathing.

EBSTEIN'S PEARL

See section on milia (p. 144).

Tongue

CYSTS AND DIMPLES

During development the thyroid develops from an area along the tongue and migrates down the thyroglossal tract in the neck to its final position. Remnants of the thyroglossal tract can present as cysts and dimples. If a cyst is sufficiently large to cause problems with feeding or respiration, consideration should be made as to whether or not the cyst contains thyroid tissue before it is removed.

TONGUE-TIE (ANKYLOGLOSSIA)

This is a term used to describe a condition in which the frenulum of the tongue is attached too far forward. It may not interfere with either feeding or speech and intervention is not always necessary but division of the frenulum may be arranged.

Ears

Absence

Absence of ears is a rare finding requiring referral to the ENT surgeon, plastic surgeon and audiologist.

Abnormal shape

Dysmorphic ears may occur as a result of a syndrome, for example Treacher Collins's syndrome (see p. 176), may be developmental or may be familial. Any baby with such an abnormality should be referred to the ENT surgeon, plastic surgeon and audiologist.

Position

Low-set ears may be indicative of a syndrome, for example Edward's syndrome (see p. 178).

Pre-auricular skin tags

Pre-auricular skin tags are not uncommon and are not always associated with abnormal hearing. If there are multiple skin tags an audiology screen should be requested. All pre-auricular skin tags are best referred to the plastic surgeon for removal.

Pre-auricular dimples

Pre-auricular dimples are more likely to be associated with abnormalities of hearing and any baby with this defect should be referred to the plastic surgeon and the audiologist.

Eyes

Discharge

Causes of discharge include infection (conjunctivitis) and blockage of the lachrymal duct. Despite the common nature of this symptom in neonates, it should be carefully monitored and appropriately investigated. If an infection is suspected because the discharge is profuse or purulent, the eye should be swabbed for bacterial and chlamydial infection and the baby should be started on topical antibiotics. Ointments are more effective in the treatment of eye infections as they remain in contact with the eye for a greater period of time.

Infection can be gonococcal, staphylococcal or chlamydial:

- *Gonococcal infection* usually manifests 2–5 days after the birth; the discharge is copious and purulent, and occurs in association with oedema of the eyelids and conjunctiva. Intensive treatment of both eyes is necessary as the condition may lead to ulceration and perforation of the eye.
- *Staphylococcal conjunctivitis* manifests 3–5 days after the birth and is less severe than gonococcal infection.
- *Chlamydial conjunctivitis* usually occurs later than gonococcal and staphylococcal conjunctivitis. Isolation of the organism requires a conjunctival scrape sample to be analysed for intracellular inclusions. It will respond to erythromycin, but untreated it can cause damage to the eye.

Confirmation of gonococcal or chlamydial infection in the neonate should be followed by counselling for the mother and her partner.

A blocked lachrymal duct usually becomes patent with time and rarely requires ophthalmic intervention to unblock it.

Ptosis

This is the term used to describe a drooping eyelid. It may be congenital. If the drooping lid covers the pupil, referral to an ophthalmologist is necessary so that vision can be accurately assessed.

Squint

This is common in babies but it is usually a transient finding that corrects itself within minutes. Epicanthic folds (see below) and a broad nasal bridge can often produce an apparent squint. Few genuine squints are detected in the neonatal period, but if the examiner is convinced that there is a persistent squint the baby is best referred to an ophthalmologist for an opinion.

Epicanthic folds

These are vertical pleats of skin that overlap the medial angle of the eye (see Figure 6.3). They are common in infants and may result in the illusion that there is a squint. They are a normal feature in the Mongoloid races and in Down's syndrome (see p. 175).

Anophthalmia

Absence of an eye can occur spontaneously or as part of a syndrome. It is usually associated with a shallow orbit, so for cosmetic reasons, and for examination of the normal eye, the baby should be referred to an ophthalmologist.

Microphthalmia

A small eye may occur as a result of congenital infection, for example rubella. It will almost certainly interfere with vision and so the baby should be referred to an ophthalmologist. It may be worth screening for evidence of congenital infection, and other features suggestive of congenital infection should be sought.

Macrophthalmia

A large eye most commonly occurs as a result of congenital glaucoma, a condition in which the drainage of fluid from the eye is obstructed, so causing a build-up of pressure in the eye. The cornea may also appear hazy in association with congenital glaucoma. Referral to an ophthalmologist should be made as a matter of urgency.

Coloboma

Coloboma of the iris appears as a sector-shaped gap. That gap may extend posteriorly to include the ciliary body and choroid. It may be isolated or part of a syndrome. Referral to an ophthalmologist is necessary.

Aniridia

Absence of the iris can occur spontaneously or in association with nephroblastoma. Referral to an ophthalmologist is necessary and the kidneys should be scanned.

Heterochromia

An iris that has different pigment may not be apparent at birth, but may develop as the eyes change from their newborn blue to their 'adult' colour.

Translucent iris

This occurs when there is reduced pigmentation of the iris, as occurs in albinism. Referral to an ophthalmologist is necessary.

White reflex (see red reflex, p. 90)

A white rather than a red reflex occurs with retinoblastoma (a retinal tumour) or scarring of the retina. The baby should be referred to an ophthalmologist for an opinion.

Cataract

A cataract is an opacity of the lens. Cataracts vary in size and may be small dot-like lesions that cause no interference with vision, or may be severe enough to produce a completely opaque lens. Some are hereditary whereas others are attributable to congenital infection (e.g. rubella) or biochemical imbalance (e.g. hypocalcaemia). The baby should be referred to an ophthalmologist to assess vision.

Neck

The neck may be shortened in association with vertebral anomalies, for example Klippel–Feil syndrome. Turner's syndrome is associated with webbing of the neck. Damage to the sternomastoid muscle results in a sternomastoid tumour, a benign swelling within the muscle, and congenital torticollis ('wry neck').

Abnormal swelling of the neck may result from a sternomastoid tumour or a cystic hygroma (a multicystic lesion of lymphatic origin). Branchial cleft remnants may present as dimples.

Limbs, including hands and feet

Palsy

When there has been a traumatic birth, particularly with shoulder dystocia, the baby may have sustained damage to its arm as a result of the accoucher delivering the posterior arm first or exerting traction to the fetal head, in an attempt to expediate the birth. Referral to an orthopaedic surgeon or a surgeon with a specific interest in this should be considered if the palsy fails to resolve within the first few weeks of birth.

- *Erb's palsy* results from damage to the fifth and sixth cervical nerve roots. It is often referred to as the 'waiter's tip position' because the elbow is extended, the arm is rotated outwards, the wrist flexed and the fingers partially closed, as if the sufferer were awaiting a discreet payment.
- *Klumpke's palsy* results from damage to the seventh and eighth cervical and first thoracic nerve roots. This palsy affects the lower half of the arm, giving rise to a limp wrist and paralysed hand.
- *Total brachial plexus palsy* results from damage to the fifth, sixth, seventh and eighth cervical and first thoracic nerve roots (i.e. the whole brachial plexus). This palsy involves paralysis of the whole arm with circulatory problems and lack of sensation (Greig 2003).

Absence or deformity

Absence of an arm can result as part of a syndrome or may be an isolated abnormality that has occurred as a result of a disruption in the sequence of development, an ischaemic event, or amputation secondary to an amniotic band. Deformity can result from those same causes or as a result of intrauterine position.

Deformity resulting from congenital absence of the fibula or radius can be associated with other abnormalities, for example low platelet count (thrombocytopenia). It can also result from congenital contractures (arthrogryposis). It should be noted that for all cases of limb deformities, other than those that are postural, early referral to an orthopaedic surgeon is essential.

Hands

Non-pitting oedema (lymphoedema) of the hands and feet is associated with both Turner's and Noonan's syndromes (see pp. 175–6). The baby should be examined carefully for other features associated with the syndromes, and blood should be collected for chromosome analysis. The lymphoedema should improve with time.

Palmar creases

Single palmar creases are associated with Down's syndrome (see p. 175), but beware because 10% of the normal population have a unilateral single palmar crease and 5% have bilateral single palmar creases.

Feet

The feet may be abnormally positioned. Talipes equinovarus describes feet that are plantarflexed (turned downwards and inwards), whereas talipes calcaneovalgus describes feet that are dorsiflexed (turned upwards and outwards).

Digits

Polydactyly

Extra digits can occur spontaneously, as a familial trait or as part of a syndrome. Enquire whether polydactyly is a familial trait; if not, examine the baby carefully for other abnormal features. Bilateral polydactyly, particularly postaxial (on the medial aspect of the hand or lateral aspect of the foot) polydactyly, is often associated with renal anomalies so arrange a renal ultrasound scan to exclude these.

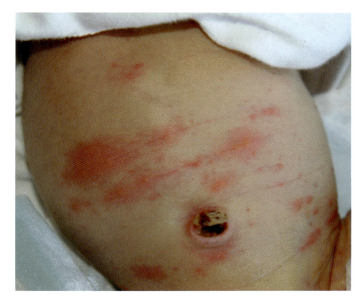

Plate 1 *Erythema toxicum*
This appears shortly after birth and is characterised by pustules on erythematous macules. They usually disappear within 2 weeks of birth and the baby remains well.

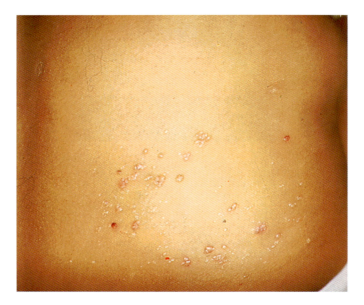

Plate 2 *Lymphangioma circumscriptum*
A collection of small vesicles that occur as a result of an abnormal collection of lymphatic channels that penetrate into subcutaneous tissues. Intervention is not usually possible.

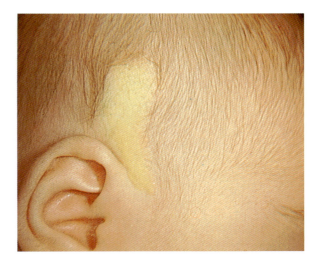

Plate 3 *Sebaceous naevus*
A yellow-brown or orange-pink skin lesion commonly on the scalp or face. The baby should be referred to a dermatologist as it may become malignant at puberty.

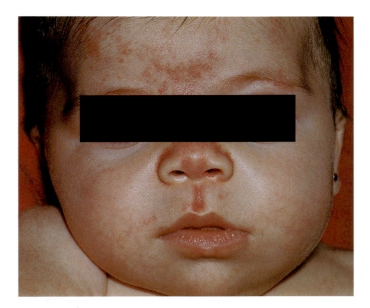

Plate 4 *Salmon patch naevus*
A faint pink patch usually found on the nape of the neck, glabella or upper eyelid. Those on the nape of the neck persist, whereas the others usually disappear.

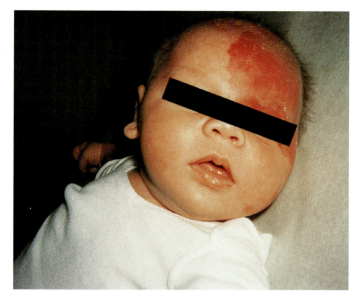

Plate 5 *Port wine stain*
A blue-purple, red or pink vascular marking that may darken with age. It can occur anywhere on the body and may be associated with certain syndromes such as Edward's, Beckwith–Wiedemann and Sturge–Weber syndromes.

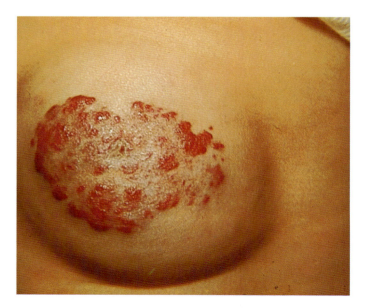

Plate 6 *Strawberry haemangioma*
At birth, this appears as a pale area with spidery blood vessels. During the first 6 months it develops into a bright red strawberry-like growth and will subsequently involute.

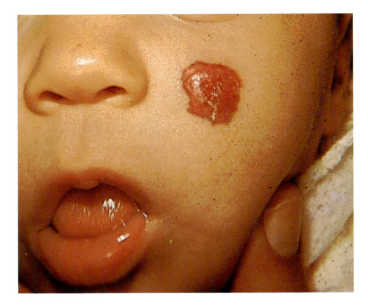

Plate 7 *Cavernous haemangioma*
This abnormal collection of blood vessels appears as a blue discolouration of the skin. It usually grows with the child. Larger lesions should be closely monitored as they may lead to haemorrhage or cause high output cardiac failure and thrombocytopenia.

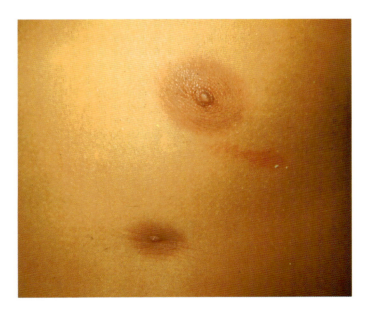

Plate 8 *Supernumerary nipple*
This additional breast tissue has as much risk of developing carcinoma as normally positioned breast tissue. It may be wise to refer to a surgeon for removal.

Radiography of the hand will reveal whether the extra digit has a bony component. If the extra digit has a bony component, refer the baby to an orthopaedic surgeon. Otherwise the anomaly can be referred to a plastic surgeon.

Syndactyly

Fusion of digits can occur spontaneously, as a familial trait or as part of a syndrome, for example Apert syndrome. Enquire whether syndactyly is a familial trait; if not, examine the baby carefully for other abnormal features.

Radiography of the hand will reveal whether the syndactyly has fusion of the bones within. If there is fusion refer the baby to an orthopaedic surgeon. Otherwise the anomaly can be referred to a plastic surgeon.

Clinodactyly

Short inward-curved little fingers can occur spontaneously, as a familial trait or as part of a syndrome, for example Down's syndrome. Enquire whether clinodactyly is a familial trait; if not, examine the baby carefully for other abnormal features. If this is the only finding, no action is necessary.

Skin

The skin may be affected by trauma, retention of secretions, hormonal instability, developmental abnormalities, congenital conditions and infection. Some of these produce similar findings and so they are grouped together by their appearances rather than their causes. Before these skin conditions are described it is necessary to understand the associated terminology (Table 7.3).

Cuts and abrasions

These are carefully observed as they may serve as portals for infection. Discovery of any injuries should always be carefully documented to avoid the potential for future dispute regarding their origin, for example iatrogenic or possible non-accidental injury.

Bruises

Bruises may result from a difficult birth or clinical interventions, for example taking blood. Most bruises are not sufficiently large to produce major problems, but as they are broken down they contribute to the bilirubin load and so to jaundice.

TABLE 7.3 The skin: glossary of terms

Term	Meaning
Erythema	Superficial reddening of the skin
Petechiae	Fine purple/red non-blanching spots
Papule	Pimple, spot, small eruption on the skin
Vesicle	Blister, fluid-filled bubble on the skin
Pustule	Pimple containing pus
Macule	Dark blemish on the skin
Naevus	Birthmark comprising raised red areas on the skin

Petechiae

These are often evident following a precipitate birth or if the umbilical cord was tight around the neck; they are usually on the face. However, they can also occur with thrombocytopenia and may be found in association with congenital infection, for example toxoplasmosis, rubella, cytomegalovirus or herpes. Each of these congenital infections is usually associated with other abnormalities, which should be considered if the diagnosis is suspected.

Milia

These are small papules, white or yellow in colour, which usually appear grouped together. They are commonly found on the face, but can occur on the body. They are caused by the retention of sebaceous gland secretions when tiny follicular ducts become plugged. An Ebstein's pearl is a milia either on the hard palate of the mouth or on the penis. They usually resolve spontaneously within the first 8 weeks of life.

Milaria

These are small vesicles with surrounding erythema that disappear when the skin cools. They are caused by blockage of sweat ducts with subsequent leakage into the epidermis.

Neonatal acne

This condition is characterised by small pustules with erythematous bases. It is caused by increased sebaceous gland activity secondary to maternal androgens and resolves with time.

Erythema toxicum neonatorum (Plate 1)

This can occur anywhere on the body very shortly after birth and is characterised by pustules on erythematous macules. They can be fleeting and at times can appear quite angry looking, but the baby remains well at all times. They usually disappear within 2 weeks of birth.

Neonatal impetigo

In neonatal impetigo vesicles or pustules appear on an erythematous base and denude and begin to crust. It is caused by staphylococcal or streptococcal infection, and the baby is usually well. It is serious and highly infectious and requires treatment with intravenous antibiotics.

Congenital herpes

In congenital herpes a vesicular eruption appears with surrounding erythema. There is usually multisystem involvement and there is a high morbidity and mortality rate. Rapid diagnosis and treatment is necessary if further progression is to be prevented. Treatment is with intravenous aciclovir.

Incontinentia pigmenti

These inflammatory vesicles develop within the first 2 weeks of life. They subsequently progress through several stages, including diffuse wart-like lesions, whorled hyperpigmentation and finally hypopigmentation in later childhood. It is found almost exclusively in girls.

Sucking blister

This is a blister without any surrounding inflammation and is the result of the fetus sucking the skin *in utero*. It resolves without treatment.

Epidermolysis bullosa

This is a group of blistering diseases differentiated from one another by histological criteria, mode of inheritance and healing capability. Blisters occur in response to varying degrees of contact and leave scarring. It is an inherited condition resulting in excessive response to trauma. Some types are associated with a high mortality rate because of complications. Meticulous skin care and urgent treatment of skin infections may reduce the degree of scarring.

Lymphangioma circumscriptum (Plate 2)

This collection of small vesicles occurs as a result of an abnormal collection of lymphatic channels that penetrate into subcutaneous tissues. No intervention is possible as surgery may be too difficult.

Erythema

NEONATAL *CANDIDA*

This yeast infection occurs on the skin, causing redness (often with satellite lesions), and in the mouth, forming a white coating, which is not easily removed by scraping. It is caused by *Candida albicans* and left untreated it can result in poor feeding or a persistent nappy rash. Treatment with topical antifungals should eradicate the fungus, but precautions should be taken to prevent reinfection, for example the breastfeeding mother must be treated and teats, nipple shields and dummies should be cleaned thoroughly.

Hypopigmentation

ALBINISM

In albinism there is reduced pigmentation of skin, hair and/or retinae. This is a genetic condition and referral to a dermatologist (and ophthalmologist if there is eye involvement) is necessary.

ASH LEAF MACULES

These are hypopigmented areas of skin with an irregular outline, best seen with a Wood's (ultraviolet) lamp. They are characteristic of a neurocutaneous syndrome called tuberous sclerosis. The condition is associated with intracardiac lesions, an abnormal cranial CT scan, a tendency to epilepsy and other skin abnormalities such as shagreen (sharkskin) patches.

Pigmentation

MONGOLIAN BLUE SPOTS

These are areas of blue-grey pigmentation, commonly found in infants of non-Caucasian parents. They are usually found over the back or buttocks, tending to fade during the first year of life, and are of no clinical significance.

CONGENITAL PIGMENTED NAEVI

These appear as pigmented plaques or papules of variable size and colour. The depth of tissue involvement may vary considerably. There is a risk of malignancy with time. The baby should be referred to a dermatologist.

CAFE-AU-LAIT SPOTS

These appear as light-brown coffee-like stains on the skin. More than six *cafe-au-lait* spots measuring greater than 1.5 cm in size suggests a diagnosis of neurofibromatosis. They are also associated with other conditions, namely tuberous sclerosis and Albright's syndrome (a condition in which there can also be fibrous dysplasia of bone, precocious puberty and facial asymmetry).

SEBACEOUS NAEVUS (OF JADASSOHN) (PLATE 3)

This has the appearance of a collection of cholesterol deposits. It is yellow-brown or orange-pink in colour and more commonly appears on the scalp or face. It may become malignant at puberty, and hence the baby should be referred to a dermatologist.

Vascular lesions

SALMON PATCH NAEVUS (PLATE 4)

This is a faint pink patch usually found on the nape of the neck, glabella or upper eyelid. Those on the nape of the neck persist, whereas the others usually disappear.

PORT WINE STAIN (PLATE 5)

This is a blue-purple, red or pink vascular marking that may darken with age. It can occur anywhere on the body. It may be associated with certain syndromes such as Edward's, Beckwith–Wiedemann and Sturge–Weber (port wine stain of the first branch of the trigeminal nerve with vascular malformations of the meninges and cerebral cortex on the same side) syndromes.

STRAWBERRY HAEMANGIOMA (PLATE 6)

At birth, this appears as a pale area with spidery blood vessels (telangiectasia). During the first 6 months it develops into a bright red strawberry-like growth. It will subsequently involute. It results from an abnormal collection of capillaries and venules. It may obstruct vision or break down and become infected.

CAVERNOUS HAEMANGIOMA (PLATE 7)

This appears as a blue discoloration of the skin. It is an abnormal collection of larger vascular elements in the skin and it usually grows with the child. It may haemorrhage or cause high output cardiac failure and thrombocytopenia.

ICHTHYOSIS

Ichthyosis is thickened, scaly, fish-like skin. It is inherited as a genetic condition. Topical agents may produce some symptomatic relief. Referral to a dermatologist may be needed.

APLASIA CUTIS

This condition is absence of the skin. It may be ischaemic in origin and it is associated with some syndromes. It usually heals spontaneously, although larger defects may require grafting.

Chest

Shape

UNDERDEVELOPED CHEST

A poorly developed chest wall may be the result of certain syndromes, for example Poland's syndrome or thoracic dystrophy (see pp. 180–1).

HYPERINFLATION

In hyperinflation the chest appears barrel shaped. It may occur as a result of a diaphragmatic hernia (a defect in the diaphragm allowing abdominal contents to pass into the chest) or air trapping as occurs in meconium aspiration syndrome.

ASYMMETRY

The normal chest wall is usually symmetrical. For causes of asymmetry see Table 7.1 (p. 120).

Nipples

WIDELY SPACED NIPPLES

Widely spaced nipples are associated with chromosomal abnormalities, for example Turner's syndrome (see p. 175). It is wise to check the number of chromosomes if other features suggest a syndrome.

ADDITIONAL NIPPLES (PLATE 8)

Any associated breast tissue has as much risk of developing carcinoma as normally positioned breast tissue. It may be wise to refer to a surgeon for removal.

Cardiovascular system

Colour (see pp. 115–25)

Heart rate and rhythm

The heart rate may be reduced with heart block, maternal medication or maternal systemic lupus erythematosis. It may be increased with thyrotoxicosis, maternal medication and supraventricular tachycardia (SVT).

FEMORAL PULSES/PULSE VOLUME

Femoral pulse volume may be reduced or absent with left ventricular outflow obstruction, e.g. coarctation of the aorta, and poor left ventricular function, e.g. hypoplastic left heart. The pulse volume may also be reduced with sepsis.

APICAL IMPULSE

The apical impulse is the impulse felt when the hand is laid over the apex of the heart. It is normally palpable in the fifth intercostal space in the mid-clavicular line. For causes of a displaced apical impulse see Table 7.1 (p. 121).

HEAVES/THRILLS

Left sternal heave is evidence of right ventricular hypertrophy. Upper left parasternal systolic thrill occurs with pulmonary stenosis. Lower left parasternal systolic thrill occurs with a ventricular septal defect.

Heart sounds

FIRST HEART SOUND

This may be quieter with a complete atrioventricular septal defect as the valve components may not close efficiently.

SECOND HEART SOUND

The aortic component of the second heart sound may be louder with aortic coarctation. The pulmonary component of the second heart sound may be louder and may precede the aortic component with pulmonary hypertension.

THIRD HEART SOUND

This may be heard when left ventricular filling is increased, for example persistent ductus arteriosus and ventricular septal defect.

FOURTH HEART SOUND

This is audible at the apex with aortic stenosis or systemic hypertension. It is audible over the right ventricle with pulmonary stenosis or pulmonary hypertension.

MURMURS

An ejection systolic murmur is caused by flow through one of the outflow valves, that is, pulmonary or aortic. It does not necessarily indicate stenosis of that valve as it can occur with the increased blood flow through the pulmonary valve that occurs with an atrial septal defect.

A *pansystolic murmur* represents escape of blood from a ventricle into an area of low pressure, as occurs with an incompetent atrioventricular (mitral or tricuspid) valve or a ventricular septal defect. An *early diastolic murmur* represents incompetence of the outflow valves, that is, aortic or pulmonary valves. A *mid-diastolic murmur* represents turbulent blood flow through the atrioventricular valves (mitral or tricuspid) as occurs when they are stenosed. A *presystolic murmur* may occur when turbulence of blood at one of the atrioventricular valves (mitral or tricuspid) results during atrial contraction.

Oxygen saturation

This is routinely assessed in some maternity units. Any settled air-breathing baby aged more than 2 hours that does not achieve a post-ductal fractional saturation of at least 95% on initial examination should have the measurement repeated 1–2 hours later. If the second measurement is less than 95% the baby should be referred for echocardiography as there is a strong possibility that the baby may have a cardiac anomaly (Richmond *et al.* 2002).

Respiratory system

Colour (see pp. 115–25)

Respiratory effort and rate

RECESSION

This is the term used to describe in-drawing of the chest wall below (subcostal) and between (intercostal) the ribs. It occurs as a result of the increased work of breathing. For causes see Table 7.1 (p. 121).

GRUNTING

This is more of a 'moaning' noise heard at the end of each expiration. It represents air being exhaled against a partially closed glottis in an effort to increase the pressure in the terminal airways and so keep them inflated. For causes see Table 7.1 (p. 122).

Respiratory pattern

For causes of apnoea, tachypnoea and grunting see Table 7.1 (p. 122).

Air entry

This is usually symmetrical, but because of the relatively close proximity of the larger airways to the chest wall the breath sounds may sound bronchial in nature, i.e. like those heard over the larynx or over consolidated tissue. This, combined with the relatively small surface area of the neonate's chest, makes it more difficult to differentiate between normal tissue and consolidated tissue by auscultation alone. Added sounds, for example crackles (crepitations), wheeze (rhonchi) and stridor, are significant. For causes of unequal air entry and additional sounds see Table 7.1 (p. 123).

Abdomen

Colour

A red or dusky abdomen is not normal. It may indicate an overly inflamed bowel. It may also indicate ascending infection from the umbilicus. The baby should be examined carefully, paying particular attention to the presence of temperature instability, vomiting, jaundice, abdominal discomfort and passage of faeces. For causes of a discoloured abdomen see Table 7.1 (p. 123).

Shape

SCAPHOID ABDOMEN

An in-drawn or sunken abdomen is referred to as scaphoid. It can betray the presence of a diaphragmatic hernia (a defect in the diaphragm allowing abdominal contents to pass into the chest). The baby should be examined carefully, paying particular attention to whether there is any respiratory compromise. Under these circumstances urgent chest and abdominal radiography should be requested to exclude this diagnosis.

DISTENDED ABDOMEN

The presence of a distended abdomen may indicate an underlying obstruction. Pay particular attention to whether there is any vomiting, jaundice or abdominal discomfort and whether the baby has passed faeces.

In the presence of these symptoms urgent abdominal radiography should be requested to exclude a diagnosis of obstruction. Radiography may not be confirmatory and so the opinion of a paediatric surgeon may be required.

PRUNE BELLY

This condition is rare. It is the result of lax abdominal muscles and is often associated with congenital megaureter (big ureter), renal anomalies and bilateral undescended testes in the male. Renal ultrasound will detect small dysplastic (abnormally developed) kidneys and congenital megaureter. The opinion of a paediatric surgeon or nephrologist will be required.

EPISPADIAS AND BLADDER EXTROPHY

Epispadias is a condition in which the urethra is abnormally formed and is often associated with bladder extrophy. The defect can affect both sexes. In the male the urethra appears to be open on the upper surface of the penis. In the female the urethra opens onto the lower abdominal wall. Epispadias usually communicates proximally with a bladder that is open to the anterior abdominal wall. This defect is also associated with abnormal formation of the bones of the symphysis pubis and requires specialised surgery that only a few centres can offer.

Organomegaly

Hepatomegaly and splenomegaly

For potential causes see Table 7.1 (p. 123).

Enlarged kidney(s)

This condition usually occurs secondary to hydronephrosis (dilatation of the ureter by urine), but can occur as a result of abnormal development, for example cystic dysplastic (abnormally formed) kidney or nephroblastoma (renal tumour).

An urgent ultrasound scan is needed, and further information may be obtained by performing a micturating cystourethrogram (MCUG). A paediatric surgical opinion may be necessary for marked hydronephrosis and is definitely required for nephroblastoma.

Large bladder

This is most obvious when there is bladder outlet obstruction, e.g. posterior urethral valves, or a neuropathic bladder, i.e. one with a faulty nerve supply. Examine the baby carefully, paying particular attention to the urinary stream, the spine and the neurological examination.

An urgent ultrasound scan is needed, and further information may be obtained by performing an MCUG. A paediatric surgical opinion will be necessary for posterior urethral valves and may be necessary for a neuropathic bladder.

Masses

Abdominal mass is the term used for a unidentified swelling felt in the abdomen. The site of any mass is often a good indicator of its source; however, confusion can arise when an organ develops elsewhere and its natural course of migration is disturbed. Masses most commonly palpated in the abdomen include:

- hydroureter;
- obstructed bowel;
- ovarian cysts;
- horseshoe kidney.

Abdominal radiography and ultrasound will provide valuable information about the mass, but contrast studies may also be required, as may the assistance of a paediatric surgeon.

Tenderness

This is difficult to assess in a baby, but when there is obvious discomfort associated with palpation this usually indicates underlying pathology, for example ischaemia, obstruction, trauma, etc. Check the maternal notes for evidence of a traumatic birth. Examine the baby carefully looking for evidence of temperature instability, vomiting, jaundice, passage of faeces, and trauma.

An infection screen may be indicated in conjunction with radiological investigation, for example ultrasound and radiography.

Groin swelling

A hernia is felt as a swelling. It often contains bowel. Most are found in the groin and are reducible, i.e. can be gently pushed back from where they came. If it is not reducible the baby will require urgent referral to the paediatric surgeon. A reducible hernia will require an outpatient referral to the paediatric surgeon.

Absent femoral pulses

See Chest, Table 7.1 (p. 121).

Male genitalia

Scrotum

APPEARANCE

A scrotum may be small with no rugae because there may never have been testes within it. Examine the baby carefully to detect ectopic or maldescended testes. Absence of both testicles should alert the examiner to the fact that the baby's sex may be indeterminate. This will necessitate careful examination of the baby and further investigations, e.g. chromosome analysis.

BIFID

Occasionally the scrotum develops as a bifid (split) structure. The baby should be examined carefully to confirm that there are testes present in each half of it and that the rest of the genitalia are normal.

SWELLING

A large scrotum may be the result of a hydrocoele. A hydrocoele is a swelling in the groin or scrotum containing fluid. It can be distinguished from a hernia by shining a bright light source directly onto the overlying skin – a hydrocoele will transilluminate (glow). Hydrocoeles do not usually require any intervention, unless they cause compression of the testicle, but should resolve spontaneously.

PIGMENTATION

Pigmentation of the scrotum is common in babies born to parents who are not white. For other causes see Table 7.1 (p. 124).

DISCOLORATION

Discoloration of the scrotum occurs with a neonatal torsion (twist) of the testis; the testicle is usually painful in this condition. Ultrasound may provide useful information, but referral to a paediatric surgeon may be necessary to exclude the condition.

Testes

UNILATERAL UNDESCENDED TESTICLE

In the absence of one testicle, the groin on the side of the absent testicle should be carefully palpated as the testicle may not have completed its descent from the posterior abdominal wall. It is also prudent to palpate just below the groin as the testicle may have descended abnormally to that area (see below).

If a testicle is undescended it may yet complete its descent and so it is worthwhile notifying the GP rather than arranging a formal surgical follow-up. It must be made clear to the parents that the testicle should be descended by the age of 1 year or surgical intervention will be necessary to locate the testicle in the scrotum.

MALDESCENDED TESTICLE

If a testicle has descended abnormally and has come to lie in the femoral triangle (the area directly below the groin) this should be discussed with a paediatric surgeon.

BILATERAL ABSENCE OF THE TESTES

Absence of both testicles should alert the examiner to the fact that the baby's sex may be indeterminate. This will necessitate careful examination of the baby and further investigations. These investigations will include ultrasound of the pelvis and abdomen to locate female reproductive organs and/or undescended testes and chromosome analysis. The baby should then be discussed with an endocrinologist and a paediatric surgeon in the light of the examination findings and results of the investigations.

Penis

SIZE

The penis size may vary considerably, but if it still appears to be small when compared with centile charts for stretched penile length the baby should be examined carefully. It may be worth discussing the baby with an endocrinologist.

SHAPE

In the condition known as chordee the penis is tethered to the scrotum on its underside. This results in the penis being curved. It can result in problems with erection later in life. The baby should be referred to a paediatric surgeon for advice regarding the possible need for correction.

Hypospadias is a term used to describe an abnormal shape to the penis. It may be merely a hooded appearance to the foreskin or an abnormality of shape in association with a meatus located abnormally either on the glans or on the underside of the penis. An isolated hooded foreskin requires no intervention, but a malpositioned meatus may result in a poor urinary stream and may be associated with abnormalities of the urethra and kidneys. A renal ultrasound may be required, as may surgery, and so the baby should be referred to a paediatric surgeon. The parents should be discouraged from having the baby circumcised as the foreskin is used in the repair procedure.

This may be the result of a narrow meatus or posterior urethral valves. Examine the baby carefully, paying particular attention to the foreskin and its opening. If ballooning of the foreskin occurs during urination, the baby should be discussed with a surgeon. An urgent renal ultrasound will not show posterior urethral valves, but it may show resultant obstruction; an MCUG is necessary to exclude the diagnosis of posterior urethral valves.

Female genitalia

Labia

APPEARANCE

Pigmentation of the labia is common in babies born to parents who are not white. For other causes see Table 7.1 (p. 124).

SIZE

If the labia are large, this may alert the examiner to the fact that there could be testes within them. They may also appear large in small-for-dates and preterm babies.

MASSES

There may be palpable testes within what appear to be the labia. Ultrasound of the pelvis and abdomen will help to identify female reproductive organs, if present.

Vagina

TAGS

These are often found in this area. They do not usually cause any problems and most can be left as they become relatively smaller with time.

BLEEDING

Pseudo-menstruation can occur as a result of withdrawal from maternal hormones. It usually begins within the first 48 hours of the birth and may persist for up to 6 days. At times it can be quite heavy, but there are never frank clots present, although there may be some mucus present.

Clitoris

SIZE

This is usually not particularly large but in preterm or small-for-dates babies it can appear large. If there are concerns about its size the baby should be examined carefully to confirm gender, taking particular care to check for testes.

Urinary meatus

POSITION

This is placed between the clitoris and the vaginal orifice. If urine is seen to dribble from any other point then a diagnosis of ectopic urethra should be considered and the baby should be examined carefully and discussed with a paediatric surgeon.

MICTURITION AND STREAM

It is unusual in the female baby to have any obstruction to the passage of urine. They are certainly not prone to posterior urethral valves.

Anus

Patency

A clearly imperforate anus requires urgent referral to the paediatric surgical team. In some cases of imperforate anus the anus may seem to be perforate but there may be an obstruction at a higher level than is evident on external examination. If this is suspected then referral to a paediatric surgeon is necessary.

Position of the anus

An anteriorly placed anus is commonly associated with problems. If the anus appears to be anteriorly placed but the baby is not having any difficulties passing meconium then an outpatient referral to the paediatric surgical team may be all that is necessary.

Meconium leaking from sites other than the anus is indicative of a fistula. The presence of a fistula is an indication for urgent referral and investigation.

Delayed passage of meconium

Delay in the passage of meconium beyond 24 hours should alert the practitioner to the possibility of problems such as Hirschprung's disease or imperforate anus, but it may also be delayed if the baby passed meconium *in utero*. Check the notes for evidence of meconium-stained liquor. Examine the baby carefully, paying particular attention to feeding, vomiting and abdominal distension.

If the baby has severe abdominal distension and vomiting within hours of the birth, meconium ileus should be suspected, a symptom present in 20% of neonates with cystic fibrosis (Hull and Johnston 1993). If there is associated abdominal distension, radiography may reveal evidence of obstruction, but it may be necessary to refer the baby to a paediatric surgeon

Hips

Positive Ortolani's/Barlow's manoeuvre

These results are suggestive of a congenital dislocation of the hip and the baby should therefore be referred to an orthopaedic surgeon.

Asymmetry

Asymmetry may reveal an underlying congenital dislocation of the hip. Examine the baby carefully, paying particular attention to the result of Ortolani's manoeuvre (see p. 105). Refer to an orthopaedic surgeon if Ortolani's manoeuvre is positive.

Reduced range of movement

This may be indicative of a congenitally dislocated hip. Pay particular attention to skin creases and the result of Ortolani's manoeuvre. Refer to an orthopaedic surgeon if Ortolani's manoeuvre is positive.

Spine

Deformity

This may be the result of a hemivertebra or abnormal growth of the spine. This can occur spontaneously or in association with various syndromes. Examine the baby carefully, paying particular attention to the neurological examination. Discuss the findings with an orthopaedic surgeon.

Overlying marks or defects (including sacral dimples)

Such marks may indicate an underlying abnormality, for example spina bifida may be associated with an overlying tuft of hair or a naevus. Examine the baby carefully. Pay particular attention to the neurological examination. A sacral dimple with a visible base is insignificant; however, if the base cannot be visualised, consider radiography and ultrasound examination of the affected area. Discuss the baby with a neurosurgeon if findings are positive.

Central nervous system

Abnormal behaviour (see pp. 125–31)

Abnormal behaviour may include:

- a high-pitched cry;
- a lethargic baby;
- an irritable baby;
- a jittery baby;
- hypo- and hypertonia;
- asymmetrical reflexes;
- an inability to suck or feed.

Evidence of any of the above may indicate a neurological problem. Cranial ultrasound examination may reveal an underlying abnormality. The baby may need to be discussed with a paediatric neurologist and investigated further. See Table 7.1 (pp. 117–18) for further details.

Abnormal cry

See Behaviour, Table 7.1 (p. 117).

Checklist

When the examination is complete, the examiner must make sure that all points referred to in the checklist at the end of Chapter 6 have been completed.

Specific abnormalities

Cardiac

Cyanotic congenital heart disease

TRANSPOSITION OF THE GREAT ARTERIES (FIGURE 7.4)

The aorta normally arises from the left ventricle and the pulmonary artery from the right ventricle, but in this condition the aorta arises from the right ventricle and the pulmonary artery from the left ventricle. *In utero* this does not pose a problem because pulmonary blood flow is small and there is movement across the patent ductus arteriosus and the patent foramen ovale, but once the baby is born and these two channels close two parallel circulations develop through the heart rather than one continuous circulation. The baby becomes increasingly cyanosed and heart failure develops. There is usually no associated murmur, but the second heart sound may be noted to be louder than usual because of the close proximity of the aorta to the anterior chest wall.

A chest radiograph may show a slightly enlarged heart with a narrow pedicle in association with heart failure. An electrocardiogram (ECG) is usually not useful at this stage. Pulse oximetry in the air-breathing settled baby, measuring the post-ductal fractional oxygen saturation in one foot after the age of 2 hours, should suggest a cardiac abnormality, but a cardiac ultrasound scan will confirm the diagnosis.

The baby requires urgent treatment with prostaglandin to re-open the duct, and referral to a cardiologist for balloon septostomy and subsequent corrective surgery.

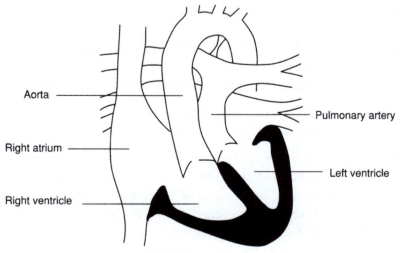

FIGURE 7.4 Transposition of the great arteries

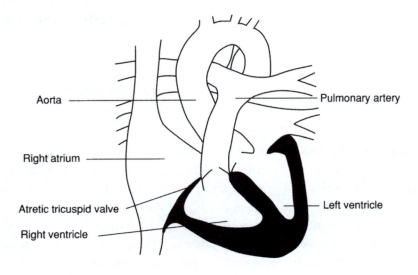

Aorta

Pulmonary artery

Right atrium

Atretic tricuspid valve

Right ventricle

Left ventricle

FIGURE 7.5 Tricuspid atresia

TRICUSPID ATRESIA (FIGURE 7.5)

This condition results in cyanosis because of reduced blood flow to the lungs. Deoxygenated blood returning to the heart can only circulate by crossing through a patent foramen ovale. It then mixes in the left atrium with oxygenated blood from the lungs and is passed into the left ventricle where it is pumped out to the body via the aorta. Pulmonary circulation is dependent on there being either a ventricular septal defect (allowing blood to move from the left ventricle to the right and out through the pulmonary artery) or a patent ductus arteriosus present (allowing the passage of blood from the aorta to the pulmonary artery). There may not be a murmur, but there is only a single second heart sound.

A chest radiograph shows oligaemic lung fields and an ECG shows a superior axis and left axis deviation.

The baby requires urgent referral to a cardiologist for assessment.

PULMONARY ATRESIA (FIGURE 7.6)

This baby is dependent upon a patent ductus arteriosus to maintain pulmonary circulation. As the duct closes, the baby becomes increasingly cyanosed. There is usually no heart murmur, but there is only a single second heart sound.

A chest radiograph shows an enlarged right atrium in association with oligaemic lung fields. An ECG shows right ventricular hypertrophy.

The baby requires urgent treatment with prostaglandin and referral to a cardiologist for assessment.

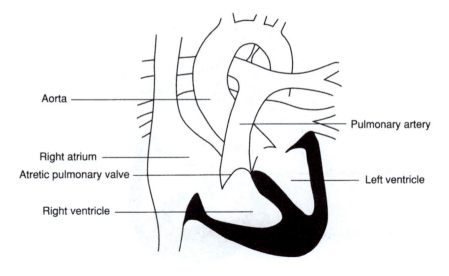

FIGURE 7.6 Pulmonary atresia

FALLOT'S TETRALOGY (FIGURE 7.7)

This condition does not always present in the neonatal period. It consists of a ventricular septal defect, an over-riding aorta, stenosis of the pulmonary valve or infundibulum and subsequent right ventricular hypertrophy. The baby is usually pink but with time develops cyanosis, which can become exacerbated as a result of spasm of the pulmonary infundibulum. At this time a pulmonary stenosis murmur may be audible.

A chest radiograph shows a concave left heart border in association with oligaemic lung fields.

The baby requires urgent referral to a cardiologist. Treatment is usually surgical, but spasm may be prevented by the use of propranolol.

TOTAL ANOMALOUS PULMONARY VENOUS DRAINAGE

This is rare but can be mistaken for lung disease in a neonate. Abnormal drainage of the pulmonary veins to one of several places results in obstruction of the vessel(s) with subsequent pulmonary venous congestion. The baby is tachypnoeic and cyanosed. There may be a loud pulmonary second sound because of the pulmonary hypertension that develops as a result of the congestion.

Sometimes the chest radiograph is diagnostic, but the opinion of a cardiologist is usually required to confirm the diagnosis.

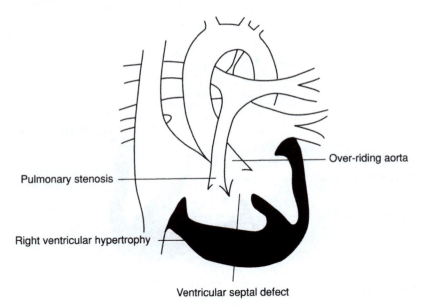

Over-riding aorta

Pulmonary stenosis

Right ventricular hypertrophy

Ventricular septal defect

FIGURE 7.7 Fallot's tetralogy

EBSTEIN'S ANOMALY

In this rare condition the baby may present with neonatal cyanosis. The right atrium is enlarged at the cost of the size of the right ventricle. The tricuspid valve is also abnormal and incompetent. The baby is cyanosed and there are additional heart sounds as well as the systolic murmur of tricuspid incompetence.

A chest radiograph shows a large globular heart ('wall to wall heart') with right atrial enlargement and oligaemic lung fields. An ECG shows tall P waves. The opinion of a cardiologist is usually required to confirm the diagnosis.

Acyanotic congenital heart disease

VENTRICULAR SEPTAL DEFECT (FIGURE 7.8)

This is the commonest of all congenital heart defects. It may be associated with other cardiac anomalies. It can occur in the membranous portion of the septum or in the muscular part. In the neonatal period these defects may be asymptomatic and there may not even be a murmur audible. In the larger defects, as the pulmonary vascular resistance falls, the flow across the defect (from left to right) increases, the lower left sternal pansystolic murmur develops, and heart failure ensues.

A chest radiograph shows an enlarged heart and pulmonary plethora. A cardiac ultrasound scan will detect the defect.

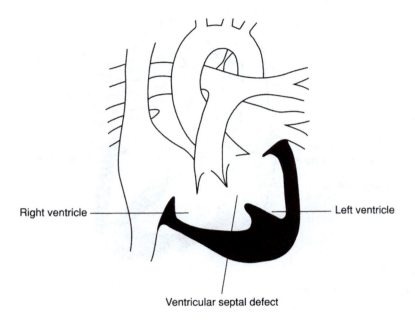

FIGURE 7.8 Ventricular septal defect

The baby should be referred to a cardiologist for assessment; the urgency of referral depends on how well the baby is. Depending on the size and position of the defect, the baby may require urgent surgery or delayed surgery or the defect may close spontaneously.

ATRIAL SEPTAL DEFECT (FIGURE 7.9)

This defect is the result of failure of the atrial septum to develop correctly. If the defect is low down it may involve the insertion of the mitral valve resulting in a cleft and incompetence. If there is mitral incompetence there may be an apical pansystolic murmur.

A chest radiograph shows cardiomegaly and pulmonary plethora. An ECG shows left axis deviation and may show an RSR pattern in V_2 (anyone unfamiliar with ECGs should refer to a standard ECG textbook for further explanation).

The baby requires referral to a cardiologist for confirmation of the diagnosis and arrangements need to be made for early correction of the defect.

ATRIOVENTRICULAR CANAL DEFECT (FIGURE 7.10)

This is an extension of the atrial septal defect causing an ostium primum defect, but involving the ventricular septum in addition to the atrial septum. The defect also involves both atrioventricular valves resulting in incompetence

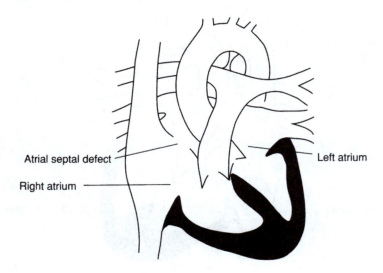

FIGURE 7.9 Atrial septal defect

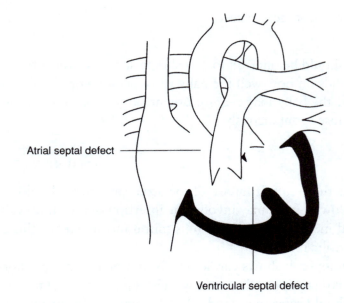

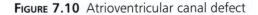

FIGURE 7.10 Atrioventricular canal defect

of both. The apical impulse is displaced because of cardiac enlargement. In the initial neonatal period there may not be a murmur, but as pulmonary vascular resistance falls a murmur develops and the baby develops heart failure.

The chest radiograph shows marked cardiomegaly and pulmonary plethora, and the ECG has a superior axis.

The baby requires assessment by a cardiologist. Heart failure may be controlled by the use of diuretics, but a repair of the defect is required if complications are to be avoided.

This is a relatively common heart lesion. It may present with heart failure in the neonatal period if the ductus is large. There is a wide pulse pressure; the apical impulse is displaced because of cardiac enlargement and there is a pulmonary systolic murmur. There may also be hepatomegaly and tachypnoea due to heart failure.

The chest radiograph shows cardiomegaly and pulmonary plethora. ECG is often not helpful in the neonatal period.

Treatment with diuretics will control the heart failure and the duct may close in response to treatment with indomethacin, but it may be necessary to refer the baby for surgical ligation of the ductus.

Obstruction to outflow

Narrowing of the pulmonary outflow tract can occur at different levels. Whatever the level, if the stenosis is severe is will present shortly after birth with cyanosis due to shunting of blood across the foramen ovale, and right-sided heart failure. There is usually a pulmonary systolic murmur audible and a right ventricular heave is palpable.

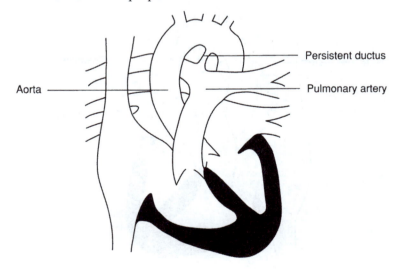

FIGURE 7.11 Patent ductus arteriosus

A chest radiograph may show an enlarged right atrium and right ventricle. An ECG shows right atrial and right ventricular hypertrophy. The baby requires referral to a cardiologist for assessment.

COARCTATION OF THE AORTA (FIGURE 7.12)

Narrowing of the descending aorta can occur at any point but most commonly occurs close to the ductus arteriosus, distal to the left subclavian artery. Depending on the degree of coarctation, the baby may have few signs or may present in a collapsed state once the ductus closes. The one important thing in identifying a coarctation is the absence of femoral pulses, although these may be present whilst the ductus remains patent if the coarctation is pre-ductal in position. There may be a murmur, which is best heard between the scapulae.

A chest radiograph may show cardiomegaly, but a cardiac ultrasound scan will identify the lesion, especially as the duct closes. A duct-dependent coarctation should respond to prostaglandin and requires urgent referral to a cardiologist for assessment.

Coarctation of the aorta is associated with Turner's syndrome, and other defects of the arch of the aorta are associated with other chromosomal anomalies, for example DiGeorge sequence with or without hypocalcaemia.

HYPOPLASTIC LEFT HEART

A diagnosis of hypoplastic left heart is sometimes made antenatally during the anomaly ultrasound scan, but if it is not detected antenatally it usually presents

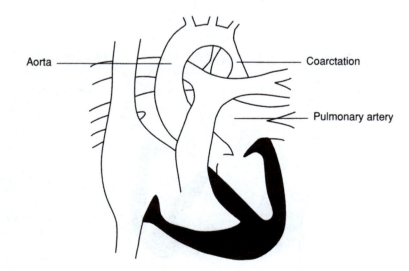

Aorta — Coarctation

— Pulmonary artery

FIGURE 7.12 Coarctation of the aorta

within days of the birth. It is thought to result from an antenatal aortic outflow tract obstruction. This produces antenatal left ventricular hypertrophy, which subsequently results in a poorly functioning left ventricle postnatally. An unanticipated hypoplastic left heart presents as a baby with severe cardiac failure, i.e. tachypnoea, hepatomegaly, poor perfusion, etc.

A chest radiograph will show heart failure, but a cardiac ultrasound is diagnostic. The baby should be referred to a cardiologist as a matter of urgency.

Respiratory

Respiratory distress syndrome

This condition is caused by reduced production of lung surfactant and occurs as a result of prematurity, hypoxia, acidosis and maternal diabetes. There is also a condition called congenital surfactant deficiency. Surfactant deficiency makes it more difficult for the lungs to expand and increases the work of breathing. The baby becomes cyanosed, has subcostal recession and tachypnoea, and may have an expiratory grunt.

Chest radiography shows a classical ground glass appearance. Blood gas analysis will show a respiratory acidosis and hypoxia. This will become more marked and often requires treatment with respiratory support, surfactant and intravenous fluids. As the condition is difficult to distinguish from congenital pneumonia it is usual for the baby to be commenced on intravenous benzylpenicillin.

The natural progression of the disease is for it to begin to resolve any time up to 72 hours of age, although this can vary. In some babies the illness can be so severe that death is inevitable.

Congenital pneumonia

This infection is commonly associated with prolonged rupture of the membranes. The responsible organism is not always isolated, but the organism most commonly causing pneumonia is the group B streptococcus. Other organisms causing congenital pneumonia include *Escherichia coli*, *Listeria monocytogenes* and staphylococci. As with respiratory distress syndrome, the baby is cyanosed with tachypnoea and recession. There may also be an expiratory grunt.

A chest radiograph will show the pneumonia and an arterial blood gas will show hypoxia and respiratory acidosis. The baby requires treatment with antibiotics and may require intravenous fluids and respiratory support.

Pneumothorax

A pneumothorax is not uncommon but depending on the size of the pneumothorax the symptoms may vary in severity. The baby is usually tachypnoeic. There may be recession, cyanosis, grunting and unequal air entry. If the pneumothorax is sufficiently large, the chest will transilluminate with a cold light source.

A baby who is relatively well but who has respiratory symptoms can be radiographed and the findings will be characteristic. In a baby who has collapsed as a result of a pneumothorax there will not be sufficient time to arrange a chest radiograph, but the presence of the pneumothorax can be confirmed by transillumination and immediate action can be taken. A small pneumothorax will resolve spontaneously, but a larger symptomatic one will require draining.

Choanal atresia

This may be bilateral or unilateral. A bilateral atresia will present early on with cyanosis and even obstructive apnoea. A unilateral atresia may come to light at a later stage. Unilateral atresia can be confirmed by obstructing each nostril in turn. When the patent nostril is obstructed, the baby will behave like a bilateral atresia.

Insertion of an oropharyngeal airway (if tolerated) will alleviate the obstruction temporarily, but the baby will require urgent referral to an ENT surgeon. CT scan usually confirms the atresia.

Gastrointestinal

Oesophageal atresia and tracheo-oesophageal fistula

There are many different combinations of abnormalities of the oesophagus and trachea, but the main one is a blind-ending upper oesophagus in association with a communication between the lower oesophagus and the trachea. Oesophageal atresia may be diagnosed antenatally by the presence of polyhydramnios. Postnatally, the diagnosis is often made following choking or cyanotic episodes as a result of the baby being unable to swallow his own secretions.

If the diagnosis is suspected the first priority is to protect the airway by commencing frequent suction of the pharynx. The baby should be carefully examined to exclude other abnormalities (anal, cardiac, skeletal and genitourinary). The diagnosis can be confirmed by attempting to pass a wide-bore (FG 10 or 12) radio-opaque nasogastric tube. Inability to pass the tube into the stomach is strong evidence for the presence of atresia, although presence of a tracheo-oesophageal fistula with no oesophageal atresia may allow a nasogastric tube to be passed; therefore, diagnosis should be confirmed by radiography. The presence of gas in the bowel, despite an atresia, is confirmation that there is a tracheo-oesophageal fistula.

The baby requires urgent referral to a paediatric surgeon for division of the fistula and repair of the atresia, which may be difficult if the two ends of the oesophagus are not close to each other. Other abnormalities should not be forgotten and should be dealt with appropriately.

Diaphragmatic hernia

This hernia may be diagnosed antenatally, but some may present at birth as a baby who is difficult to resuscitate, or even later with tachypnoea. The majority are left-sided and so are associated with displacement of the heart sounds and apical impulse to the right. There is also reduced air entry on the left and a scaphoid abdomen.

The baby should be resuscitated and then examined carefully for other abnormalities. A chest radiograph will confirm the diagnosis. Once confirmed, a large-bore nasogastric tube should be inserted into the stomach and allowed to drain freely to avoid accumulation of air and its passage into the hernia, which would compromise breathing further. There is often associated pulmonary hypoplasia and the baby may require ventilation.

The baby requires urgent referral to a paediatric surgeon who is experienced in dealing with the anomaly.

Duodenal atresia

This is a relatively high obstruction and as such its presence may not be recognised early on because it is less likely to cause marked abdominal distension and may not necessarily be associated with bile-stained vomiting. Any distension that occurs is restricted to the epigastrium, but may be associated with visible peristalsis.

The baby should be examined carefully as the abnormality is associated with Down's syndrome. An abdominal radiograph or ultrasound will show the classical 'double bubble' of duodenal atresia.

The baby requires urgent referral to a paediatric surgeon for further investigations and repair of the lesion.

Imperforate anus

Like oesophageal atresia, an imperforate anus is not always apparent, and there are numerous anatomical variations. The anomaly may be apparent when the baby is first examined, but it may become apparent only when the baby develops abdominal distension or fails to pass meconium. The 'high' imperforate anus is the least obvious and may or may not be associated with a recto-vaginal or recto-vesical fistula. The 'low' anomaly may merely consist of a membrane covering the anus.

The baby should be examined carefully as the anomaly may be part of a collection of abnormalities. An abdominal radiograph will show intestinal obstruction and the absence of gas in the rectum. The baby will require urgent referral to a paediatric surgeon for further investigation and treatment.

Gastroschisis

In gastroschisis a defect in the anterior abdominal wall allows the bowel to protrude through it. Unlike exomphalos there is no sac covering the bowel and this abnormality is not usually associated with other abnormalities.

The defect allows major fluid and heat loss to occur and so the exposed bowel is best covered with clingfilm to minimise this and intravenous access should be established. Urgent transfer to a paediatric surgical unit is necessary.

Exomphalos

In exomphalos abdominal contents protrude through the abdominal ring into the umbilical cord. They are covered with a transparent sac. There is a risk of heat and fluid loss and so the contents are best covered with clingfilm. There is an association with chromosomal, cardiac, gastrointestinal and genitourinary abnormalities as well as with Beckwith–Wiedemann syndrome. The baby should be examined carefully to exclude other abnormalities and the blood sugar should be monitored to exclude hypoglycaemia. It may be necessary to take blood for chromosome analysis and to arrange further investigations to exclude associated abnormalities. The baby should be referred to a paediatric surgeon for repair of the defect.

Genitourinary

Posterior urethral valves

This is a condition that affects male babies and results in obstruction to the flow of urine with hydronephrosis. It is commonly suspected antenatally by the presence of hydronephrosis on antenatal ultrasound. It can cause impaired renal function, but this may be reversible with drainage and careful attention to fluid and electrolyte balance.

The condition is confirmed by MCUG. The baby requires urgent referral to a paediatric surgeon for disruption of the valves.

Ambiguous genitalia

This condition can occur as a result of many different problems, for example chromosomal, hormonal, etc. Whatever the reason, it is important to the parents for the baby to be assigned to one or other gender as quickly as possible. However, the gender to which the baby is assigned requires careful consideration of the following three aspects:

1. *genetic sex*, i.e. chromosomal karyotype;
2. *gonadal sex*, i.e. the presence or absence of testes, which will only develop in response to the H-Y antigen;
3. *functional sex*, i.e. the usefulness of the organs present.

Check the maternal notes for evidence of family history of ambiguous genitalia or neonatal death and exposure to drugs in pregnancy. Examine the baby carefully, paying particular attention to the appearance and size of the genitalia and other abnormalities.

Blood should be taken for chromosome analysis and urea and electrolytes, plasma ACTH (adrenocorticotrophic hormone) and 17-hydroxyprogesterone levels. A pelvic ultrasound will identify the female reproductive organs, if present. Other radiological investigations may be necessary. The baby should be discussed with an endocrinologist and a paediatric surgeon as a matter of urgency.

Hypospadias

The majority of these anomalies are glandular or coronal and merely require the practitioner to confirm that the baby is passing urine adequately. More severe forms may be associated with other abnormalities, for example renal, intersex, etc.

The baby should be examined carefully. If the hypospadias is more severe, a renal ultrasound should be arranged. The parents of a baby with hypospadias that is not glandular should be encouraged to avoid having the baby circumcised as the foreskin may be required to repair the abnormality. The baby should be referred to a paediatric surgeon for repair of the abnormality.

Epispadias

This condition affects boys more frequently than girls. In the male with epispadias the urethra is a strip of mucosa on the dorsum of the penis. In the female there is a double clitoris and the urethra is split dorsally.

The baby should be examined carefully to exclude other abnormalities. A renal ultrasound should be requested. The baby requires urgent referral to a paediatric surgeon.

Bladder extrophy

This condition affects boys more frequently than girls. There is complete epispadias, exposure of the bladder mucosa on the anterior abdominal wall and division of the symphysis pubis.

Careful examination should take place to exclude further abnormalities. A renal ultrasound should be requested. The baby requires urgent referral to a paediatric surgeon.

Musculoskeletal

Some babies with skeletal dysplasias may present difficulties at the birth requiring resuscitation. Pulmonary hypoplasia may result from external compression as a result of a small chest cage, as seen in the lethal condition thanatophoric dwarfism.

Achondroplasia

This is a dominantly inherited condition, but it may also occur as a result of a spontaneous mutation. There is a normal-size trunk in association with short limbs and a large head. There may be hydrocephalus.

If either parent has achondroplasia then that is the likely diagnosis. Skeletal radiographic changes are characteristic and a cranial ultrasound will exclude hydrocephalus. Paediatric follow-up is necessary, although the outcome is usually good.

Osteogenesis imperfecta

This may result in multiple fractures of the long bones and ribs antenatally with subsequent deformities.

The abnormality may be diagnosed *in utero*, but postnatally the diagnosis can be confirmed by radiography of the bones. The baby requires referral to an orthopaedic surgeon.

Specific syndromes

The practitioner should ensure that whenever a syndrome has been confirmed the parents are referred to a geneticist for counselling.

Down's syndrome (trisomy 21)

Down's syndrome results from additional genetic material from chromosome 21. The common form (94%) consists of the addition of a complete chromosome 21 to the chromosome complement, i.e. trisomy 21, but less common forms are the result of partial duplication of genetic material from chromosome 21. The incidence of Down's syndrome was 1 in 660 newborns (Jones 1997) but this will have reduced with the introduction of antenatal screening and selective termination of some fetuses. The majority of cases can be diagnosed clinically, but chromosome analysis allows confirmation of any less obvious cases. The clinical features most commonly found at birth include:

- craniofacial: flat facial profile, upward-slanting eyes;
- eyes: inner epicanthic folds, Brushfield spots (speckling of the iris);
- neuromuscular: hypotonia;
- hands and feet: relatively short metacarpals and phalanges, clinodactyly (inward curving) of the fifth finger, a wide gap between the first and second toes, single palmar crease and abnormal dermatoglyphics.

There may be an associated cardiac anomaly (most commonly complete atrioventricular septal defect or ventricular septal defect) and gastrointestinal anomaly (duodenal atresia or Hirschprung's disease).

Blood should be taken for chromosome analysis. An ECG may assist in excluding certain cardiac abnormalities, but referral to a paediatric cardiologist is advisable. The baby will require paediatric follow-up, as there will be developmental delay.

Turner's syndrome

Turner's syndrome results from the absence of a sex chromosome. The best known karyotype is XO, in which there is complete absence of a sex chromosome, but the syndrome can result from partial deletion of a sex chromosome or from a mosaic genotype in which there is absence of sex chromosomes in some cells and not in others. The estimated incidence is 1 in 2000 live-born females (Turner Syndrome Support Society 2009). The clinical features most commonly found at birth include:

- growth: small stature;
- hands: lymphoedema, narrow hyperconvex nails;
- skeletal: cubitus valgus (outward angle of arm from elbow);
- thorax: widely separated nipples;
- neck: webbing of the neck, low posterior hairline;
- facies: relatively small mandible.

There may be an associated cardiac anomaly (most commonly bicuspid aortic valve and coarctation) and renal anomalies (horseshoe kidney) and there will be short stature and infertility.

Blood should be taken for chromosome analysis. A renal ultrasound scan may exclude horseshoe kidney. Referral to a paediatric cardiologist is advisable to exclude coarctation of the aorta. The baby will require paediatric follow-up as developmental delay is common, and the input of a paediatric endocrinologist will also be required.

Noonan's syndrome

This consists of phenotypical features of Turner's syndrome in a male baby with cryptorchidism (bilaterally impalpable testes). It usually occurs sporadically, but apparent autosomal dominant inheritance has been documented and a gene for the disorder has been mapped. The clinical features most commonly found at birth include:

- skeletal: cubitus valgus;
- thorax: shield chest and pectus excavatum or pectus carinatum;
- neck: webbing of the neck, low posterior hairline;
- facies: relatively small mandible, hypertelorism;
- genitalia: small penis, cryptorchidism.

The most commonly associated cardiac abnormality is pulmonary valve stenosis. There is also an increased incidence of coagulation and platelet defects.

Blood should be taken for chromosome analysis and molecular genetics. Referral to a paediatric cardiologist is advisable. The baby will require paediatric follow-up.

Treacher Collins's syndrome (mandibulofacial dysostosis)

This is an autosomal dominant condition, although it can occur sporadically. In some cases there is an association with a particular gene mutation. The clinical features most commonly found at birth include:

- craniofacial: malar hypoplasia, mandibular hypoplasia, cleft palate, downward slanting eyes;
- ear: malformation of auricles;
- eye: lower lid coloboma (full thickness deformity), absence of lower eyelashes.

The condition can be so severe that it causes problems with airway patency. There is often associated deafness. In the first instance the priority is to maintain the airway if there are any difficulties with this. Take a look at both parents – either may have the condition. Blood should be taken for molecular genetic analysis. The baby will require an audiology assessment and it may be necessary to refer him to an ENT surgeon. Paediatric follow-up will be necessary.

Pierre Robin's syndrome

Pierre Robin's syndrome comprises:

- craniofacial: small jaw (micrognathia), a mid-line cleft palate and a protruding tongue (glossoptosis).

These features can occur to a greater or lesser degree. The main problem is that of airway obstruction secondary to the tongue falling back and obstructing the oropharynx. The baby can also experience problems with feeding.

This will require referral to an ENT surgeon, speech therapist and orthodontic surgeon. The small jaw may also require referral to a craniofacial team.

Apert's syndrome (acrocephalosyndactyly)

This is an autosomal dominant condition, but the majority of cases are sporadic. It is associated with a particular gene mutation. The clinical features most commonly found at birth include:

- craniofacial: short anteroposterior diameter, high forehead, flat occiput, craniosynostosis (premature fusion of suture) of the coronal suture, cleft palate, downward slanting eyes;
- hands and feet: syndactyly (webbing).

Blood should be taken for molecular genetic analysis. The premature fusion of sutures puts the growing brain at risk of compression so it is necessary to refer the baby to a neurosurgeon. Syndactyly will require referral to an orthopaedic surgeon. The baby will also require paediatric follow-up as mental deficiency is common.

Crouzon's syndrome (craniofacial dysostosis)

This is an autosomal dominant condition with variable expression, but it can occur sporadically. It is associated with a mutation of the same gene responsible for Apert's syndrome. The clinical features at birth include:

- craniofacial: ocular proptosis, hypoplasia of the maxilla, high forehead, craniosynostosis (coronal, lambdoid and sagittal).

Blood should be taken for molecular genetic analysis. It will be necessary to refer the baby to a neurosurgeon as progressive intracranial hypertension will develop if the craniosynostosis is not treated. The baby will also require paediatric follow-up.

Patau's syndrome (trisomy 13)

Patau's syndrome occurs in 1 in 5000 births (Jones 1997). It results from trisomy for all or most of chromosome 13. The majority (82%) of these babies die within the first month of life. The clinical findings at birth include:

- craniofacial: microcephaly, narrow palpebral fissure, depressed saddle nose, high philtrum, cleft lip, cleft palate;
- ears: low set, abnormal helices;
- eyes: microphthalmia, colobomata of iris;
- hands and feet: flexion and overlapping of the fingers, polydactyly;
- genitalia: cryptorchidism (undescended testes).

Cardiac abnormalities such as ventricular septal defect, patent ductus arteriosus and atrial septal defect are common. Incomplete development of the forebrain is a common finding.

Examine the baby carefully. Blood should be taken for chromosome analysis. The baby will require referral to a paediatric cardiologist to exclude a cardiac anomaly. He will also require a cranial ultrasound scan and paediatric follow-up.

Edward's syndrome (trisomy 18)

Edward's syndrome had an incidence of 1 per 5000 newborn babies (Simpson 2004), although with antenatal screening and selective termination this incidence will have been reduced. It results from trisomy for all or most of chromosome 18. The majority (90%) of those affected die within the first year of life. The clinical features found at birth include:

- growth: intrauterine growth retardation;
- craniofacial: micrognathia, short palpebral fissure, epicanthic folds, narrow bifrontal diameter, prominent occiput;
- ears: low set;
- hands: flexion deformity of the fingers;
- genitalia: cryptorchidism.

Cardiac abnormalities are common and include ventricular septal defect, atrial septal defect and patent ductus arteriosus. Mental deficiency is common.

Examine the baby carefully. Blood should be taken for chromosome analysis. The baby will require referral to a paediatric cardiologist to exclude a cardiac anomaly. He will also require paediatric follow-up.

Cri du chat syndrome

This results from a partial deletion of chromosome 5. Approximately 85% of cases occur spontaneously. Clinical findings at birth include:

- growth: low birth weight;
- craniofacial: microcephaly, occular hypertelorism (increased distance between the eyes), downward slanting eyes, facial asymmetry;
- ears: low set;
- hands: single palmar crease, abnormal dermatoglyphics;
- general: cat-like cry;
- neuromuscular: hypotonia.

There also appears to be an increase in the incidence of congenital heart disease (variable abnormalities). All babies subsequently go on to develop learning difficulties.

Blood should be taken for chromosome analysis. Paediatric follow-up is essential.

Goldenhar's syndrome (hemifacial microsomia)

This syndrome results from abnormalities in the development of structures that are derived from the first and second branchial arches. Most cases occur sporadically, but there is a risk of recurrence in first-degree relatives of about 2%. Clinical features evident at birth include:

- facial: hypoplasia of malar, maxillary or mandibular region, macrostomia (wide mouth);
- ear: microtia (small ear), pre-auricular tags or pits.

There are often associated abnormalities of the vertebrae (hemivertebrae) and abnormalities of the eye such as microphthalmia or dermoids. There is also an increased incidence of cardiac abnormalities (ventricular septal defect, patent ductus arteriosus, Fallot's tetralogy and coarctation), and renal anomalies (ectopic kidneys, reflux and dysplasia) are also common.

A renal ultrasound scan will exclude most of the associated renal anomalies. A paediatric cardiologist will detect cardiac anomalies. Cosmetic surgery will probably be necessary as will assessment of hearing. Paediatric follow-up should be arranged.

Möebius sequence (sixth and seventh nerve palsy)

This occurs as a result of one of four different problems:

1. hypoplasia or absence of the nerve nuclei in the brain;
2. destructive degeneration of the nerve nuclei in the brain;
3. peripheral nerve involvement;
4. myopathy.

It most commonly occurs sporadically, but in some cases it can be familial with an autosomal dominant inheritance. The clinical features at birth include:

- facial: expressionless facies (facial palsy), micrognathia (small jaw).

Paediatric follow-up is required as some cases have associated learning difficulties.

Poland's syndrome

In this condition the fullness of the upper part of the chest is lacking as a result of hypoplasia or absence of the pectoralis major muscle. There may be associated anomalies, e.g. hypoplasia/absence of the nipple and areola, distal limb hypoplasia (syndactyly/oligodactyly) and renal anomalies. A renal ultrasound should be requested.

Thoracic dystrophy

The chest appears elongated and thin. Respiratory compromise may be sufficient to cause respiratory distress and even death.

Beckwith–Wiedemann syndrome

Clinical findings at birth include:

- abdominal: exomphalos;
- growth: the baby is usually large for dates;
- metabolic: there are often problems with glucose metabolism;
- ears: there is a characteristic linear skin crease on the ear lobe.

The baby's blood sugar should be monitored carefully and hypoglycaemia should be dealt with appropriately. A renal ultrasound should be performed as there is a risk of nephroblastoma. The baby will require paediatric follow-up.

DiGeorge sequence

Clinical findings at birth include:

- immunological: T-cell defects;
- cardiac: aortic arch abnormalities, e.g. coarctation;
- metabolic: hypoparathyroidism leading to hypocalcaemia.

Calcium levels should be monitored closely and hypocalcaemia treated appropriately. Because of the risk of an aortic arch anomaly the baby should be referred for an urgent cardiac opinion. The baby will also require immunological investigations and paediatric follow-up.

Summary

We have explored the nature and initial management of some of the major abnormalities that may be suspected or discovered during the first examination of the newborn. Thankfully most babies are born perfectly healthy. However, the practitioner examining the baby must acknowledge that her care during this examination has the potential to make a valuable contribution to the future health and well-being of the neonate. The next chapter focuses on professional accountability and effective clinical practice in relation to the first examination of the newborn.

Self-test

1. A baby is said to be 'jittery'. What conditions might you consider to be the cause?
2. What do you think is the most common cause of facial asymmetry?
3. What concerns might you have for a baby who has an extensive port wine stain involving the scalp?
4. What feature of a ptosis would concern you?
5. What might be the cause of a poorly palpable femoral pulse?
6. What condition might you think of in a baby with respiratory distress and a scaphoid abdomen?
7. What cardiac conditions would cause a baby to be cyanosed?
8. What diagnoses need to be considered in an apparently male baby with undescended testicles?
9. How would you confirm unilateral choanal atresia?
10. What antenatal finding might lead you to suspect the presence of oesophageal atresia and how would you confirm it?

Activities

- Think about how you would proceed with the examination of, discussion about and referral of a baby who on first glance appears to have Down's syndrome but whose parents do not appear to be aware of this.
- Consider some different congenital abnormalities, e.g. tongue-tie, bladder extrophy, accessory digits. Compile a list of specialists in your area to whom you might refer a baby with a problem. Is your local paediatric team (medical or surgical) able to manage such problems or would the baby require management further afield?
- Consider the agencies that you might need to contact before discharging a baby home if the baby is:
  - jaundiced;
  - hypotonic and requiring tube feeds;
  - known to have an abnormal antenatal ultrasound scan showing a dilated renal pelvis;
  - at risk of abuse;
  - heard to have a heart murmur at 48 hours of age.

Resources

- Association of Breastfeeding Mothers. Support and advice for women who want to breastfeed. http://www.abm.me.uk/
- Birthmark Support Group. Advice for professionals, patients and carers. http://www.birthmarksupportgroup.org.uk/
- Congenital Heart Information Network. Information, resources and support for families, adults and professionals. http://tchin.org/
- Down's Syndrome Association. Support and information for parents and professionals. http://www.downs-syndrome.org.uk/
- Turner Syndrome Support Society. Advice for carers. http://www.tss.org.uk/
- Systematic review: Knowles *et al*. (2005). http://www.hta.ac.uk/1207

Chapter 8   **Accountability and effective care**

Introduction

Although the purpose of the first examination of the newborn is to confirm normality, there are some potentially life-threatening conditions, such as some forms of congenital heart disease, that are not evident in the first 24 hours of the baby's life and which therefore would not be detected (MacKeith 1995). When the practitioner performing this clinical examination of the baby is new to the role, it is likely that she will have some concerns about the risk of litigation in the event of an abnormality being missed. For example, what is the legal position of a practitioner who does not detect a congenital condition in a baby during the first examination of the newborn? It is therefore essential that this examination is performed with competence and an appreciation of the practitioner's accountability. Practitioners must recognise and acknowledge the responsibility that they carry (Michaelides 1997).

The aim of this chapter, therefore, is to acknowledge the role and responsibilities of practitioners who undertake the first examination of the newborn and to remind them of their professional, legal and employment accountability. The main focus of the second half of the chapter is to illustrate how the practitioner can take positive steps to increase the effectiveness of the first examination of the newborn, and it includes issues such as gaining and maintaining competence. Before these concepts are explored it is important that practitioners appreciate the role of the various members of the multidisciplinary team who have had responsibility for the first examination of the newborn.

Acknowledging professional responsibilities and boundaries

The role of the midwife includes 'to examine and care for the newborn infant' (Nursing and Midwifery Council 2004: 37) and this skill is taught within the pre-registration midwifery programmes. This initial examination is undertaken shortly after the birth to confirm normality and identify readily apparent physical abnormalities such as cleft lip or spina bifida. It does not, however, encompass the detailed examination of the heart, lungs, eyes, abdomen or hips that a paediatrician traditionally undertakes within the first 72 hours – *the first examination of the newborn.*

For the registered nurse or midwife to undertake such an examination, a course of education, supervised practice and assessment of competence must be undertaken. Such an adjustment to the scope of professional practice, however, should only be undertaken if the following principles apply:

- patient care will be enhanced;
- existing care is not compromised;
- limits of practice are acknowledged;

- competence is maintained;
- accountability for practice is borne.

Such expansion of professional practice should be undertaken only in the full knowledge and agreement of the hospital trust's legal department, as it is the trust who will assume vicarious liability if a parent sues for damages. It should be supported by a locally agreed policy and medical colleagues should ideally be involved in all preparations for adjustments to the scope of professional practice that potentially affect them. Nurses and midwives will continue to need to access medical advice and expertise to support their daily practice, and every effort should be made to enhance the relationship rather than jeopardise it. Development of enhanced roles is an evolutionary process and it is important that they reach maturity having gone through an appropriate childhood and adolescence (Savrin 2009).

That nurses and midwives have taken on some aspects of the doctor's role is not a new concept; see for example the existence of the emergency nurse practitioner (Tye *et al.* 1988) and neonatal nurse practitioner (Honeyfield 2009). Such extensions to the scope of professional practice help facilitate the provision of client-centred care through increasing the choices available for patients, provide more continuity of care and reduce the length of time that patients wait to be seen (McKenna *et al.* 1994). Ultimately the aim of such roles is to improve the quality of care for a specific client group (McNamara *et al.* 2009).

We have explored issues relating to who undertakes the first examination of the newborn, and it is now appropriate that accountability within this role is further clarified.

Accountability

Nurses and midwives must always be able to justify the actions (or omissions) they make to reflect the position of responsibility they hold (Nursing and Midwifery Council 2008a). As such, being accountable is an integral part of clinical practice. This section will consider the concept of accountability as it applies to the professional practice of doctors, nurses, midwives and health visitors. It is necessary to consider the three components to which professionals must conform:

1. professional accountability;
2. legal accountability;
3. terms of employment.

Professional accountability

The regulatory body for nurses, midwives and specialist community public health nurses is the Nursing and Midwifery Council (NMC), and it defines the standards of conduct for these professions, exercising the powers conferred on it by the Nursing and Midwifery Order 2001. The General Medical Council (GMC) fulfils a similar remit for the medical profession.

The first examination of the newborn is not currently part of the role of *all* midwives or neonatal nurses. However, the midwife is an autonomous practitioner accountable for her practice within the bounds of normality. The activities of a midwife are defined in the European Union Midwives Directive 80/155/EEC Article 4 and presented in the *Midwives Rules and Standards* (NMC 2004). These activities include 'to examine and care for the newborn infant' (NMC 2004: 37), and the directive provides a legal framework for practitioners to develop clinical skills in this aspect of their role. When deviations from normal are detected, the midwife must refer the client to 'such qualified health professional as may reasonably be expected to have the necessary skills and experience to assist her in the provision of care' (NMC 2004: 16). This means that if she is concerned about the well-being of a baby, she should call a practitioner who can take the appropriate action and not, for example, a junior doctor on his first obstetric placement.

Criteria for professional behaviour of the registered nurse, midwife or health visitor are provided in *The Code. Standards of Conduct, Performance and Ethics for Nurses and Midwives* (NMC 2008a). This document states that 'as a professional, you are personally accountable for actions and omissions in your practice and must always be able to justify your decisions' (NMC 2008a: 1). Accountability applies to all aspects of practice in which the professional makes judgements and takes action as a result of those judgements, for example when giving analgesia to a patient in pain. The professional is answerable for the actions taken and these should always seek to promote the interests of the individual patient and the public in general. A professional should always be able to provide a sound rationale for any action taken. The midwife is further guided by the *Midwives Rules and Standards* (NMC 2004), which define her role and remit of practice.

Doctors must also recognise their professional accountability and, in the UK, this was redefined and presented in the government's White Paper *The New NHS: Modern, Dependable* (Department of Health 1997). This document introduced the concept of clinical governance through which trusts have a responsibility to ensure quality of clinical care through the implementation of risk management systems, evidence-based practice, lifelong learning and the systematic audit of clinical performance. Such activities are no longer optional but mandatory. The GMC requires doctors to adhere to the principles and values of ethical practice as detailed in the document *Good Medical Practice* (GMC 2006). Again, accountability is a strong theme.

Legal accountability

Professionals involved in the care of patients have a legal duty to care for them properly, that is, to the standard of a reasonable, competent member of that profession (the Bolam test). Failure to do so could result in a patient suing for compensation. For a person suing for compensation (the plaintiff) to be awarded damages in respect of negligent care it is their responsibility to demonstrate all of the following:

- the defendant owed a duty of care;
- the defendant was in breach of that duty of care;
- damage was reasonably foreseeable;
- the damage caused was a direct result of that breach (Dimond 2006).

It must be noted that ignorance of the law is no defence.

Duty of care

The duty of care is clearly established between a health professional and the client. It consists of those elements that constitute treatment, information giving, planning and evaluating care, documentation, supervision and ensuring a safe environment.

Breach of duty

The level at which care should be delivered has been determined through application of the Bolam test. This standard requires that professionals act in a similar manner to a colleague of equivalent status – no higher, no lower. However, when the midwife has assumed the duty of a paediatrician she should do so with the same skill as the person who would ordinarily assume that duty. On assuming that responsibility the nurse or midwife would not be able to say 'It was my first week' if she made a mistake, but should perform at the same level as the person who would normally undertake that role.

Causation

This is probably the most difficult element of establishing negligence. Even when a condition has failed to be diagnosed, it will constitute negligence only if correct diagnosis would have altered the management of care.

Symon (1998) outlines a case in which a child with congenital cataracts did not receive a diagnosis during the first examination of the newborn. However, an ophthalmologist involved in the case stated that if the condition had been detected at birth it would have made little difference to the treatment of the child as the prognosis for unilateral cataracts is extremely poor. This is not to suggest that failing to diagnose a condition is without reproach; however, it is not necessarily evidence of negligence, although failure to instigate steps to investigate a condition may be in some circumstances (Symon 1997a). Under current UK law, however, the plaintiff must show causal association between the breach of the practitioner's duty of care and the condition for which damages are being pursued.

It would be appropriate at this point to refer back to the question raised at the beginning of the chapter and apply the four principles of negligent care: What is the legal position of a practitioner who does not detect a congenital condition in a baby during the first examination of the newborn?

1. *The defendant owed a duty of care.* Clearly, by undertaking a professional role, practitioners owe a duty of care to their clients.
2. *Breach of the duty of care.* In relation to failing to detect a neonatal abnormality, for example, a practitioner would be in breach of her duty of care if:
    i. she did not gain informed consent from the parents;
    ii. she failed to take steps to identify it;
    iii. she was not using commonly accepted techniques to examine the baby;
    iv. a colleague of equivalent status would have been expected to detect it;
    v. she failed to act on a suspicion of abnormality;
    vi. she did not document her findings;
    vii. she did not communicate her findings to the parents;
    viii. she did not follow up investigations requested.

    It is clear from this list that there are many ways in which a practitioner could breach her duty of care to a client, even if she was clinically competent. It is important to ensure that none of the above apply to *your* practice. Failure to detect an abnormality that a colleague of equivalent status would also have missed does not constitute negligence.
3. *Foresight.* Is it foreseeable that a breach in the duty of care might cause harm? For example, could it be foreseen that if a practitioner did not document her findings, such as a heart murmur, and communicate them to an appropriate colleague the baby might be harmed by not receiving

prompt referral and treatment? The answer is clearly yes, harm is a reasonably foreseeable outcome of this breach of duty of care.

4. *Causation*. To gain compensation for a condition that was not detected at the first examination, the parents would be obliged to prove that detecting it earlier would have made a difference to the outcome.

Terms of employment

Practitioners have a contractual obligation to abide by the policies of the trust that employs them and to take due care in the performance of their duties. It is also expected that employees who are contracted as professionals will fulfil the required standards set by their regulatory body. The employer has a responsibility to ensure that there are safe systems in place to protect its employees from harm, such as protective clothing.

Trusts will accept liability for the actions of employees during the course of their contracted work and will therefore meet the financial costs of litigation. This is known as *vicarious liability*. It is for this reason that it is usually the trust that is named in negligence cases, even if the trust was not negligent in its duties. If the employee was negligent the employee would be in breach of the contract of employment and in law the employer would have the right to be indemnified, although this is unlikely to be pursued.

When a claim for compensation is made

Despite effective clinical care of the mother and her baby, if a congenital abnormality is identified there is a small but real possibility that parents will commence legal action. 'Clinical competence alone will not prevent claims being brought if the outcome is poor' (Capstick 1993: 10).

Parents often feel that they must do something positive for the child. It is a terrible fact for parents to face when an abnormality is discovered in a child. There is often a degree of self-blame, and in an attempt to assuage that feeling of guilt parents try to do everything left in their power to alleviate their child's suffering. Making a legal claim for compensation is one way that this phenomenon is manifested.

It is worth bearing in mind that, in England, a change in the legal aid rules in 1990 means that all claims on behalf of infants are funded by the state. Even if the practitioner was not negligent in her duties it is possible that parents, who are distressed because their baby has an abnormality, will file a claim, and the money is available to fund it. It is therefore important that there are no loopholes for the litigant's lawyer to exploit.

The legal process can be a long and protracted affair, with delays occurring at any stage along the way. The time taken from the initial request from the plaintiff's solicitor to see the case notes to a case going to court can be many years.

Although the financial cost of litigation, in terms of compensation, professional time and legal fees, is considerable, the human cost of the anguish experienced by the individuals involved in the case is immeasurable. It must be acknowledged, therefore, that action that reduces the risk of negligence claims being filed is time well spent.

Informed consent

Although the examination of the newborn is a clinical examination that is routinely performed on all neonates, consent is still required from the parents before it can be undertaken. In the context of the examination of the newborn the practitioner needs to be aware of both the legal and the professional aspects of gaining consent.

Legal aspects of gaining consent

We have already seen that professionals have a duty of care to provide information to patients, without which they are unable to make an informed choice. Ideally this information should be made available to parents before they have to make a decision, so that there is opportunity for them to ask questions and raise concerns. Unfortunately, it is often the case, particularly with non-invasive tests such as ultrasound scanning, that little attention is given to information before the event, if at all. Parents are likely to be devastated if their previously 'normal' baby is suddenly found to have a life-threatening abnormality, the diagnosis of which could have been initiated by the neonatal examination. Of course, it would be inappropriate to attempt to prepare every parent for the possibility that a major defect might be detected, but they should know that the neonatal examination is a screening procedure.

For consent to be valid it must 'be given voluntarily by an appropriately informed person who has the capacity to consent to the intervention in question' (Department of Health 2009b: 9). In this regard 'a person lacks capacity in relation to a matter if at the material time he is unable to make a decision for himself in relation to the matter because of an impairment of, or a disturbance in the functioning of, the mind or brain' (Department of Health 2005: 2). Capacity is assessed based on the individual's ability to understand and retain information, weigh up the consequences of consenting and communicate their decision (Department of Health 2009b).

It must also be acknowledged that failure to gain consent from the parents to undertake the examination of their baby could also be seen as assault in legal terms. It is also essential that the designation of the practitioner is made clear to parents. If a parent expects a procedure to be undertaken by a doctor, and has no reason to believe that it is not being undertaken by a doctor, then consent may be invalid if the procedure is then undertaken by a nurse or midwife (Martin 1997).

Professional aspects of gaining consent

In line with government policy set out in *Maternity Matters* (Department of Health 2007) maternity services are increasingly endeavouring to offer choices to women regarding the type of care they receive. To make choices, however, women need access to relevant, unbiased information in a language that is meaningful to them. Parents will need to know who you are, the options that are available, what you are going to do, and the advantages and disadvantages of the procedure.

WHO ARE YOU?

Your status and evidence of this should be clearly given to parents. Many professionals do not wear a uniform and this can be confusing for parents. The fear of abduction of babies from maternity units is a real one, and for this reason you should not attempt to remove the baby from the mother's side. When the environment is not conducive to a personal and thorough examination of the baby, parents should accompany you to a more private location. If you are a nurse or a midwife you should inform the parents that you have undertaken further education and supervised practice in order to undertake this role (Dowling *et al.* 1996).

OPTIONS AVAILABLE

Depending on the model of care that is operating within the maternity unit parents should be able to choose to see a doctor, a nurse or a midwife without being put under pressure to make one choice in particular. As a nurse or a midwife it would be very easy to say, 'You can see a doctor but you will have to wait because they are very busy on the special care baby unit, but I could see you now'. On the other hand, parents do have a right to know the facts and so it might be more appropriate to say, 'You are welcome to see a doctor if you would prefer, and I will find out for you when he or she will be available'. The reality is that most parents will opt to do what everyone else is doing, but their choice of practitioner should be a real one.

WHAT ARE YOU GOING TO DO?

The purpose and content of the examination should be clearly outlined to the parents. They should be reassured that any significant findings will be discussed with them and that they are free to ask questions during the examination. In a national survey of women's experiences of maternity care (Redshaw *et al.* 2007) 16% of women indicated that at least one member of staff did not communicate with them effectively.

ADVANTAGES AND DISADVANTAGES OF THE PROCEDURE

This is a very important aspect of gaining informed consent for a procedure. Examination of the newborn is a screening test and as such should be presented in the light of its ability to detect abnormality. Parents need to be aware that although the examination of their baby can exclude conditions such as congenital cataracts it may not detect some forms of heart disease (MacKeith 1995). The converse is also true: when a lax hip joint is detected during this initial examination it may not be evident subsequently.

Documentation of consent

In most situations verbal consent is all that is required, and the practitioner should document in the baby's notes that this has been gained. The form in which consent is gained does not increase its validity; it is the process by which it is sought that makes it safe. However, if consent is declined, trust policy may require a written declaration to be signed by the parents, to say that they have understood the purpose of the examination and the implications of declining it. In practice, this non-invasive screening test is rarely declined and is readily accepted as part of routine care.

Box 8.1 summarises the steps involved in gaining consent.

The next section focuses on how the effectiveness of the neonatal examination can be enhanced to ensure that families receive quality care.

Box 8.1 Gaining consent checklist

- Does the person have capacity?
- Is the consent given freely?
- Has the person received sufficient information?
- Do they understand what they are consenting for?
- Do they agree to the procedure?
- Is it documented in the notes that consent has been given?

Achieving and maintaining best practice

Practitioners responsible for examination of the newborn should consider the following issues in relation to their role:

- competence;
- multidisciplinary policy;
- senior professional and clinical support;
- documentation;
- systematic audit of practice.

Competence

Doctors, nurses and midwives need to address two aspects of their clinical competence to undertake the examination of the newborn: gaining competence and maintaining competence.

Gaining competence

Paediatricians who undertake the examination of the newborn are usually qualified doctors who are working for a paediatric consultant for approximately 6 months. They may go on to specialise in paediatrics or family medicine or, alternatively, use their experience to complement a career in obstetrics. A doctor undertaking this role will therefore already have considerable skill auscultating the heart, listening to the chest and palpating the abdomen in adults. The additional expertise required to care for babies will be gained by working alongside senior colleagues, by caring for sick neonates and through personal study.

For midwives and nurses to gain the extra skills to be competent to perform the full examination of the newborn it is necessary for them to undertake a post-registration programme of study that exposes the practitioner to this new sphere of practice. Originally pioneered by Stephanie Michaelides (1995), this education combines theory with practice and is available in a range of academic institutions. A practising newborn examiner and/or senior paediatrician assess clinical competence and on successful completion of the course the midwife is able to practise the new skill within the remit of the local policy and trust guidelines. As more nurses and midwives become skilled and experienced in this clinical examination they will be able to assess the competence of their peers.

Maintaining competence

The Code (NMC 2008a), which both nurses and midwives must abide by, states that, as a registered professional, the practitioner must 'take part in appropriate learning and practice activities that maintain and develop your competence and performance' (p. 7). Nurses and midwives must also fulfil their post-registration education and practice requirements (Prep) (NMC 2008b) of 35 hours of relevant learning in every 3-year registration period and 450 hours of practice. According to the *Midwives Rules and Standards* (NMC 2004: 17): 'A midwife . . . is responsible for maintaining and developing her own competence, and . . . must ensure she becomes competent in any new skills required for her practice'. Similarly, for doctors:

> You must keep your knowledge and skills up to date throughout your working life. You should be familiar with relevant guidelines and developments that affect your work. You should regularly take part in educational activities that maintain and further develop your competence and performance
>
> (GMC 2006: 12)

It is central to the practice of all health professionals that they acknowledge the limits of their own individual competence. It is important that practitioners do not run the risk of continuing to care when they are out of their clinical depth by thinking 'I ought to know this' and not seeking advice from senior colleagues because they are too embarrassed to admit that they do not know. It is difficult for senior professionals, who are often seen as the font of all knowledge, to admit to not knowing something, but it would be much more difficult to do the same in court. The remit for nurses and midwives is clearly stated in their professional code: 'you must recognise and work within the limits of your competence' (NMC 2008a: 7). Exactly the same wording is used in guidance for doctors (GMC 2006: 8).

Nurses and midwives are often in the fortunate position of staying within their specialty for a substantial length of time. This enables them to continue to build on their knowledge and expertise, which junior doctors who are moving between departments every 6 months do not have the luxury of (Denner 1995). It is a dual responsibility of practitioners to avail themselves of clinical update opportunities and of employers to enable practitioners to access them. Practitioners should keep a record of the updates they have accessed and, if locally required, the number of examinations they have undertaken.

Practitioners who perform newborn examinations should also make sure that they share this valuable learning opportunity with others. Student nurses and midwives are supernumerary and should be sought out whenever an examination is about to take place. In addition, students see a range of practitioners work and may be able to reflect with you on how the way that you work compares with the way that others work.

Multidisciplinary policy

The first examination of the newborn is not currently part of the role of all midwives or neonatal nurses. It is essential, therefore, that the midwife or nurse is supported in this expansion of her role by a locally agreed policy that clearly sets out her remit and provides definitive guidelines for referral to a paediatrician when support or guidance is required.

The process of sitting down together with fellow colleagues to construct a multidisciplinary policy is an extremely valuable one. Each professional group will gain insight into the constraints and obligations of their respective roles, and this will enhance their future working relationship.

An *example* of such a policy is shown in Box 8.2. The practitioner could also use this opportunity to familiarise herself with the information leaflet for parents that outlines the purpose and scope of the first examination of their baby. The practitioner can then reiterate these messages when seeking parental consent.

Box 8.2 Neonatal examination by a nurse or midwife (practitioner)

Introduction

Examination of the newborn is performed on all babies within the first 6–72 hours of life. It is currently performed by paediatric senior house officers, general practitioners and, increasingly, midwives and neonatal nurses. Its purpose is to exclude major congenital abnormality and reassure the parents that their baby is healthy. As the length of postnatal stay in hospital is declining, this first examination is often combined with the traditional discharge examination by the doctor and confirms the baby's fitness to go home. It is therefore an important screening procedure and health promotion opportunity.

Since the publication of the document *Changing Childbirth* (Department of Health 1993a) and subsequent government policy (Department of Health 2004, 2007, 2008) nurses and midwives are exploring ways that enable them to provide continuity of care to women and their families. Midwives, without medical input, transfer fit and healthy women to community care. Many midwives/ neonatal nurses feel that after receiving the appropriate education and clinical experience they are best placed to transfer the care of babies into the community.

Aim

To provide parents with the opportunity to have their baby examined by a neo-natal nurse or midwife who is competent in this role.

Objectives

The practitioner will:

- have a minimum of 2 years of post-registration experience;
- have successfully completed a course of preparation; and
- have access to 24-hour senior paediatric support in the event of an abnormality being either detected or suspected.

Protocol

The practitioner will:

- undertake the examination between 6 and 72 hours after the baby's birth;
- obtain informed consent from a parent;
- undertake examinations on babies that are term singletons with no known or expected anomalies;
- undertake a full medical examination of the baby in the presence of a parent informed by knowledge of the obstetric, medical and family history;
- make detailed records of the examination in the appropriate case notes;
- record any deviation from normal and inform the paediatrician, informing parents of all findings;
- decline to undertake an examination of a baby when workload pressures or other such circumstances would prevent the examination receiving the attention it requires; in such circumstances the paediatrician or general practitioner would be requested to undertake the examination;
- maintain a portfolio of their clinical updates (attend at least x hours each year);
- maintain a record of the examinations undertaken for audit purposes.

Reviewed by: (senior nurse/midwife/paediatrician)

Review date:

Senior professional and clinical support

During the course of professional practice, in every field of health care, there will be the need to consult an expert or seek a second opinion regarding a particular clinical situation. Multidisciplinary team work is vital in the provision of effective, high-quality care for the family unit (Leonard *et al.* 2004). Examining the neonate is such a situation in which sometimes confirmation of an observation, such as a suspected heart murmur, is required to ensure that the appropriate care is given. It must therefore be ensured that, when a practitioner is responsible for examining a neonate, senior paediatric support is available for advice and guidance when needed. This should be clearly documented in the protocol that the practitioner works within so that there is no confusion about who that clinician might be at any given time. Referral for advice and support when an abnormality is suspected or detected is not a weakness but a professional requirement (NMC 2008a).

Professional support is also required so that the practitioner can discuss any issues pertaining to practice, such as continuing professional development and workload pressures. In midwifery, the practitioner has the statutory right to have access to a supervisor of midwives for support and guidance. The practising midwife has 24-hour access to a supervisor of midwives, who can offer advice and information enabling the midwife to continue to provide high-quality care (NMC 2004: 27). The remit of the supervisor of midwives is to safeguard the mother and her baby by ensuring that midwives are able to maintain and develop their professional knowledge while acknowledging the limits of their competence. Although not universally available or always practised within nursing, clinical supervision is a mechanism that enables the practitioner to reflect on professional and practice issues within a supportive relationship (Royal College of Nursing 2002). Supervisors are optimally placed to understand the unique culture of the organisation in which the practitioner is working and therefore be empathetic to her needs. Practitioners should meet regularly with their supervisors not only for professional support, but also to discuss and evaluate their roles within ever-evolving health services.

Documentation

Records are a vital way in which health-care professionals communicate with each other. The nature of health-care work is such that we see many patients each day in similar circumstances, but requiring individualised care. Records help ensure that observations are communicated to colleagues, including any subsequent action taken, who was involved and when. Many maternity records are patient held and therefore the parents may have access to this information in the comfort of their own home. Just because the parents do not have a medical or legal background does not mean that their friends and relatives do not. There are some basic requirements that help make records effective:

• Do not use abbreviations unless a standard list of locally approved abbreviations accompanies each set of records. Abbreviations are open to misinterpretation and can lead to mistakes being made.
• Always date, time and sign each entry, stating your designation at least once on the record.
• Always write in black as it photocopies much more clearly should a copy be required.
• If you have requested referral, further tests or investigations ensure that they are documented and evaluated. All actions taken and advice given should be clearly written.
• It is also relevant to document circumstances that may have contributed to an inability to perform the examination adequately. Such an entry must be accompanied by a plan to deal with the situation. Table 8.1 illustrates how this might apply in practice.
• If unavoidable circumstances prevent the practitioner from returning to the baby, the situation should be explained to the mother and alternative arrangements made and documented in the case notes.
• Do not make amendments to records with correction fluid but, if necessary, score a single line throughout the text so that what is written underneath can be clearly read, write 'written in error' and sign the entry.
• When possible use language that is clear and accessible to the client so that it can be read with a minimum of translation. This will avoid confusion and fear caused by the use of jargon and technical language. Records should be written bearing in mind that the patients have access to all written records about themselves. They should therefore not contain any material that might be subjective, offensive or irrelevant. In ideal circumstances records should be made in front of parents so that they have a full knowledge of what observations have been documented.

TABLE **8.1** An example of a written entry in the notes

Date, time	Record	Signature	Designation
01/02/10, 10.40 hours	Unable to auscultate the heart as baby Smith was crying Plan: repeat examination this afternoon. Mother and midwife Jones informed	Jane Smith	Midwife
01/02/10, 15.20 hours	Baby Smith calm and re-examined Normal heart sounds heard. Mother informed, fit for transfer home	Jane Smith	Midwife

It cannot be emphasised too strongly how important clear, concise records are; further detail is provided in the document *Record Keeping: Guidance for Nurse and Midwives* (NMC 2009). Excellence in record keeping is central to proactive risk management. The existence of accurate, contemporaneous records may actually prevent a case ever coming to court. A decision on whether a case should be thrown out or pursued is often made after a plaintiff's solicitor writes to the hospital trust outlining a possible claim and asking for the case notes to be disclosed. There is a professional duty to keep such records and failure to do so may lead to the assumption that the care also failed to come up to scratch. A useful aspect to bear in mind when considering record keeping is the maxim that 'if it is not documented it did not happen'.

Detailed patient records are an investment for the future because the child who is damaged in the perinatal period has up to 21 years in which to file a claim (i.e. 18 years to become an adult and then 3 years of knowledge of the injury). There is no time limit to filing a claim for a child who is brain damaged (Dimond 2006). Accurate records are therefore invaluable as many staff have difficulties recollecting a particular case (Symon 1997b). We cannot see into the future and predict which parents will file for negligence on behalf of their child. It would be almost impossible to remember the precise details of what actions were taken or what referrals were made many years after the event. Although it may seem tedious at the time to make detailed notes of such interactions, if a case is brought to court these records form an essential part of the defence.

It has been shown how clear, accurate and detailed records can assist the delivery of quality care and also act in a practitioner's defence should a negligence case be initiated. Activities such as peer review of records are an excellent means of promoting best practice and exploring ways of developing strategies for enhancing care delivery.

Systematic audit of practice

Whenever we provide clinical care it is useful to know how effective we are. Examination of the newborn is no exception and the quality of the examination should be explored, monitored and reviewed on a regular basis. This is particularly important because the examination can potentially take place in a range of settings, for example in the home, hospital or community clinic/children's centre. It can also be undertaken by a range of professionals, for example midwives, neonatal nurse and paediatricians/GPs. Also, it can be undertaken at any time between 6 and 72 hours after birth, with the potential for different outcomes at different time points.

Audit is 'the systematic and critical analysis of the quality of clinical care' (Department of Health 1993b: 2). Through the implementation of clinical governance in the UK NHS following the publication of *The New NHS: Modern, Dependable* (Department of Health 1997), clinical audit has become an integral part of health-care provision. Audit involves identifying what is best practice, setting standards and then comparing practice against those standards. It is a dynamic process through which changes can be recommended and then subsequent care re-audited, and thus the cycle continues.

There are many aspects of the examination of the newborn process that can be audited to ensure that quality of care is continually improved. Donabedian (1966) suggested three aspects of care that, through their examination, can assist the practitioner to enhance quality issues. These are structure, process and outcome (see Table 8.2).

Audit identifies where systems are working well and where there is room for improvement. Thus completing the audit cycle involves making changes, and it is therefore important that the people whom the change will effect are involved at the beginning of any audit project. Planning should include all members of the multidisciplinary team and managers who might be responsible for implementing any of the recommendations. Individuals who will be required to make the changes should be involved in the decisions about how they can be achieved.

One method for examining the quality of care that is given is peer review. Asking another examiner to observe your work is an opportunity to receive constructive feedback about your performance. As independent practitioners, examiners rarely have the occasion to learn from each other through direct observation and if this process can be built into a regular quality review it can be invaluable.

Another method for providing practitioners with feedback about their work is video recording an examination. It can be a daunting prospect, but the camera does not lie. To see yourself not picking up on cues from the parents, forgetting to introduce yourself properly or avoiding eye contact can be a powerful tool in the quest for quality care improvement. Parental consent must

TABLE 8.2 Donabedian's dimensions of quality

Criteria	Characteristics	Example in practice
Structure	Resources required	Policies, skills, equipment
Process	Actions undertaken	Gaining consent, documentation, examination
Outcome	Desired effect	Patient satisfaction, no detectable abnormalities missed

be obtained, explaining how you would like to use the video, for example for personal reflection or sharing with a group or conference.

In summary, the audit cycle involves the following stages:

- identify key stakeholders;
- examine best practice and set standards;
- compare current practice against these standards by collecting data;
- analyse data and compare against standards;
- present findings to key stakeholders;
- agree and plan appropriate changes;
- implement changes;
- re-audit practice.

Summary

This chapter has given readers an insight into how their professional and legal accountability affect their role when undertaking the first examination of the newborn. There are many ways in which the practitioner can enhance the effectiveness of the examination, thus minimising the risk of mistakes being made and negligence suits being filed.

It is a privilege to be with women and their families at this special time in their lives. Every possible care should be taken to ensure that as health-care professionals we make a positive contribution to the experience of the birth of their baby.

Self-test

1. What is meant by 'professional accountability'?
2. Describe the four requisite components of clinical negligence.
3. When might a practitioner be in breach of their duty of care?
4. What is meant by the term 'vicarious liability'?
5. Who is responsible for ensuring that a newborn examiner is competent to practice?
6. What constitutes 'valid consent'?
7. Identify eight requirements of effective record keeping.
8. In what circumstances should a practitioner refer a baby to a senior colleague?
9. What are the advantages of involving the multidisciplinary team in the development of policy?
10. What are the stages of the audit cycle?

Activities

- Locate your trust's policy on examination of the newborn. When was it created and who was involved? How many examinations do you think each practitioner should undertake in a year to maintain their skills?
- Find out what opportunities are available for newborn examiners to maintain and update their skills, both nationally and locally. Where is this documented and who is responsible for monitoring this?
- How and when are the outcomes of the neonatal examination audited where you work? Who is involved? Are women's views collated and fed back so that the service can continually improve?

Resources

- Department of Health. Key consent documents. http://www.dh.gov.uk/en/Publichealth/Scientificdevelopmentgeneticsandbioethics/Consent/Consentgeneralinformation/index.htm
- Care Quality Commission. Report of record keeping. http://www.cqc.org.uk/newsandevents/newsstories.cfm?cit_id=35295&FAArea1=customWidgets.content_view_1&usecache=false
- NHS Litigation Authority. *Clinical Negligence Scheme for Trusts (CNST)*. http://www.nhsla.com/Claims/Schemes/CNST/
- Parliamentary and Health Service Ombudsman. *Changes to the NHS Complaints System*. http://www.ombudsman.org.uk/news/hot_topics/changes_nhs_complaints_system.html
- General Medical Council. Core guidance for doctors. http://www.gmc-uk.org/guidance/index.asp
- National Clinical Audit Advisory Group. http://www.dh.gov.uk/ab/NCAAG/index.htm
- Nursing and Midwifery Council (NMC). Publications and standards relevant to maintaining safe and effective clinical practice. http://www.nmc-uk.org/aSection.aspx?SectionID=12

Appendix 1 **Useful addresses**

Action on Smoking and Health (ASH)
First Floor, 144–145 Shoreditch High Street, London, E1 6JE
Tel: 020 7739 5902
Fax: 020 7729 4732
http://www.ash.org.uk/ash_home.htm

Alcoholics Anonymous
PO Box 1, 10 Toft Green, York, YO1 7NJ
Tel: 0845 769 7555
http://www.alcoholics-anonymous.org.uk/

Association for Children with Hand or Arm Deficiency (REACH)
Reach Head Office, PO Box 54, Helston, Cornwall, TR13 8WD
Tel: 0845 130 6225
Fax: 0845 130 0262
http://www.reach.org.uk

Association for Improvements in the Maternity Services (AIMS)
Tel: 0300 3650 663
http://www.aims.org.uk

Association for Spina Bifida and Hydrocephalus (ASBAH)
42 Park Road, Peterborough, Cambs, PE1 2UQ
Tel: 0845 450 7755
Fax: 01733 555985
Email: helpline@asbah.org
http://www.asbah.org/

Baby Life Support Systems (BLISS)
9 Holyrood Street, London, SE1 2EL
Tel: 020 7378 1122
Fax: 020 7403 0673
http://www.bliss.org.uk

BM The Birthmark Support Group
London, WC1N 3XX
Tel: 0845 045 4700
http://www.birthmarksupportgroup.org.uk/

Body Positive
http://bpkent.users.netlink.co.uk/net.html

British Institute for Brain Injured Children
Knowle Hall, Knowle, Bridgwater, Somerset, TA7 8PJ
Tel 01278 684060
Fax: 01278 685573
Email: info@bibic.org.uk
http://www.bibic.org.uk/

British Heart Foundation
Greater London House, 180 Hampstead Road, London, NW1 7AW
Tel: 020 7554 0000
Email: internet@bhf.org.uk
http://www.bhf.org.uk/

British Pregnancy Advisory Service
Tel: 0845 730 4030
http://www.bpas.org/

Brook Advisory Centres
Brook, 421 Highgate Studios, 53–79 Highgate Road, London, NW5 1TL
National office tel (admin): 020 7284 6040
Fax (admin): 020 7284 6050
http://www.brook.org.uk

Caesarean Support Network
55 Cooil Drive, Douglas, Isle of Man, IM2 2HF
Tel: 01624 661269

Cleft Lip and Palate Association (CLAPA)
Tel: 020 7883 4883
http://www.clapa.com/

Cry-sis
BM Cry-sis, London, WC1N 3XX
Helpline: 0845 122 8669
http://www.cry-sis.org.uk/

Cystic Fibrosis Trust
11 London Road, Bromley, Kent, BR1 1BY
Tel: 020 8464 7211
Fax: 020 8313 0472
Email: enquiries@cftrust.org.uk
http://www.cftrust.org.uk/

Cystic Hygroma and Haemangioma Support Group (CHHSG)
55 Jewel Walk, Bewbush, Crawley, RH11 8BH
Tel: 01293 571545

Diabetes UK
Macleod House, 10 Parkway, London, NW1 7AA
Tel: 020 7424 1000
Fax: 020 7424 1001
Email: info@diabetes.org.uk
http://www.diabetes.org.uk/

Disfigurement Guidance Centre
PO Box 7, Cupar, Fife, KY15 4PF
Tel: 01337 870281
Fax: 01337 870 310
http://www.timewarp.demon.co.uk/dgc.html

Down's Syndrome Association
The Langdon Down Centre, 2A Langdon Park, Teddington , Middlesex, TW11 9PS
Tel: 0845 230 0372
Fax: 0845 230 0372
Email: info@downs-syndrome.org.uk
http://www.downs-syndrome.org.uk/

DrugScope
Prince Consort House, Suite 204 (2nd floor), 109/111 Farringdon Road, London, EC1R 3BW
Tel: 020 7520 7550
Fax: 020 7520 7555
Email: info@drugscope.org.uk
http://www.drugscope.org.uk/

Dystrophic Epidermolysis Bullosa Research Association (DebRA)
Debra House, 13 Wellington Business Park, Dukes Ride, Crowthorne, RG45 6LS
Tel: 01344 771961
Fax: 01344 762661
Email: debra@debra.org.uk
http://www.debra.org.uk/

Foresight: Association for the Promotion of Preconceptual Care
178 Hawthorn Road, Bognor Regis, West Sussex, PO21 2UY
Tel: 01243 868001
Fax: 01243 868180
Email: emailus@foresight-preconception.org.uk
http://www.foresight-preconception.org.uk/

Foundation for the Study of Infant Deaths
11 Belgrave Road, London, SW1V 1RB
Tel: 020 7802 3200
Email: office@fsid.org.uk
http://fsid.org.uk

Gingerbread (association for one parent families)
255 Kentish Town Road, London, NW5 2LX
Tel: 020 7428 5400
Fax: 020 7485 4851
Email: info@gingerbread.org.uk
http://www.gingerbread.org.uk/portal/page/portal/Website

Herpes Viruses Association (HVA)
41 North Road, London, N7 9DP
Tel: 0845 123 2305
Email: info@herpes.org.uk
http://www.herpes.org.uk/

Help the Hospices (hospice information)
Hospice House, 34 Britannia Street, London, WC1X 9JG
Tel: 0870 903 3903
http://www.helpthehospices.org.uk

La Leche League of Great Britain
PO Box 29, West Bridgford, Nottingham, NG2 7NP
Tel: 0845 456 1855
http://www.laleche.org.uk/

MAMA Meet a Mum Association
54 Lillington Road, Radstock, BA3 3NR
Tel: 0845 120 3746
http://www.mama.co.uk/

Maternity Action
2–6 Northburgh Street, Finsbury, London, Middlesex, EC1V 0AY
Tel: 020 7490 7639
http://www.maternityaction.org.uk/

National Childbirth Trust
Tel: 0300 3300 770
http://www.nctpregnancyandbabycare.com/home

UK National Eczema Society
Hill House, Highgate Hill, London, N19 5NA
Tel: 020 7281 3553
Email: info@eczema.org
http://www.eczema.org/

Meningitis Trust
Fern House, Bath Road, Stroud, Glos, GL5 3TJ
Tel: 01453 768000
Helpline: 0800 028 1828
http://www.meningitis-trust.org/

National Stepfamily Association
3rd Floor, Chapel House, 18 Hatton Place, London, EC1N 8RU
Tel: 020 7209 2460
Fax: 020 7209 2461

Parentline Plus
520 Highgate Studios, 53–79 Highgate Road, Kentish Town, London, NW5 1TL
Tel: 0808 800 2222
http://www.parentlineplus.org.uk/

Pre-eclamptic Toxaemia Society (PETS)
c/o Dawn James, Rhianfa, Carmel, Caernarfon, Gwynedd, LL54 7RL
Tel: 01286 882685
Email: dawnjames@clara.co.uk
http://www.pre-eclampsia-society.org.uk/

Royal National Institute for Deaf People (RNID)
19–23 Featherstone Street, London, EC1Y 8SL
Tel: 0808 808 0123
Email: informationline@rnid.org.uk
http://www.rnid.org.uk/

Royal National Institute of Blind People (RNIB)
105 Judd Street, London, WC1H 9NE
Tel: 020 7388 1266
Fax: 020 7388 2034
Helpline: 0303 123 9999
Email: helpline@rnib.org.uk
http://www.rnib.org.uk/Pages/Home.aspx

Samaritans
The Upper Mill, Kingston Road, Ewell, Surrey, KT17 2AF
Tel: 020 8394 8300
Fax: 020 8394 8301
Helpline: 08457 90 90 90
http://www.samaritans.org/

Sands (stillbirth and neonatal death society)
28 Portland Place, London, W1N 4DE
Tel: 020 7436 7940
Fax: 020 7436 3715
Helpline: 020 7436 5881
Email: support@uk-sands.org
http://www.uk-sands.org/

Scope
6 Market Road, London, N7 9PW
Tel: 020 7619 7100
Helpline: 0808 800 3333
http://www.scope.org.uk/

Sense (national deafblind and rubella association)
101 Pentonville Road, London, N1 9LG
Tel: 0845 127 0060
Email: info@sense.org.uk
http://www.sense.org.uk/

Sickle Cell Society
54 Station Road, Harlesden, London, NW10 4UA
Tel: 020 8961 7795
Fax: 020 8961 8346
Email: info@sicklecellsociety.org
http://www.sicklecellsociety.org/

STEPS (national association for families of children with congenital abnor-
malities of the lower limbs)
Warrington Lane, Lymm, Cheshire, WA13 0SA
Tel: 01925 750271
Fax: 01925 750270
Email: info@steps-charity.org.uk
http://www.steps-charity.org.uk

Terrence Higgins Trust
52–54 Grays Inn Road, London, WC1X 8JU
Tel: 020 7812 1600
Fax: 020 7812 1601
Helpline: 0845 1221 200
Email: info@tht.org.uk
http://www.tht.org.uk/

Twins and Multiple Births Association
2 The Willows, Gardner Road, Guilford, Surrey, GU1 4PG
Tel: 01483 304442
Fax: 01483 302483
Email: enquires@tamba.org.uk
http://www.tamba.org.uk/Page.aspx?pid=195

Appendix 2 Advice for parents to reduce the risk of cot death

Place your baby on the back to sleep, in a cot in a room with you
Healthy babies placed on their backs are not more likely to choke

Do not smoke in pregnancy or let anyone smoke in the same room as your baby
Smoking in pregnancy greatly increases the risk of cot death. It is best not to smoke at all

Babies exposed to cigarette smoke after birth are also at an increased risk of cot death
Nobody should smoke in the house, including visitors. Anyone who needs to smoke should go outside

The safest place for your baby to sleep is in a cot in a room with you for the first 6 months
Do not share a bed with your baby if you have been drinking alcohol, if you take drugs, if you are a smoker or if you are very tired. Small and/or premature babies are also more at risk when bed sharing

Never sleep with your baby on a sofa or armchair
There is also a risk that you might roll over in your sleep and suffocate your baby

Do not let your baby get too hot; keep your baby's head uncovered
Babies can overheat because of too much bedding or clothing, or because the room is too hot. The room should be at about 18 degrees Celsius

Place your baby in the 'feet to foot' position in his cot
Make the covers up so that they reach no higher than the shoulders

Breastfeeding reduces the risk of cot death
Breast milk gives babies all the nutrients they need for the first 6 months of life and helps protect them from infection

Source: Adapted from Department of Health (2009c).

References

Abdel-Latif, M., Pinner, J., Clews, S., Cooke, F., Lui, K., Oei, J. (2006). Effects of breast milk on the severity and outcome of neonatal abstinence syndrome among infants of drug-dependent mothers. *Pediatrics* 117(6): e1163–9.

Adra, A.M., Mejides, A.A., Dennaoui, M.S., Beydoun, S.N. (1995). Fetal pyelectasis: is it always 'physiologic'? *American Journal of Obstetrics and Gynecology* 173(4): 1263–6.

Akhter, M.S. (1976). An unusual complication of intrapartum fetal monitoring. *American Journal of Obstetrics and Gynecology* 124(6): 657–8.

Alcock, K.M. (1992). Teenage pregnancy and sex education. *British Journal of Family Planning* 18(3): 88–92.

Alexander, J.M., Cox, S.M. (1996). Clinical course of premature rupture of the membranes. *Seminars in Perinatology* 20(5): 369–74.

Allott, H. (1996). Picking up the pieces: the post-delivery stress clinic. *British Journal of Midwifery* 4(10): 534–6.

Alroomi, L.G. (1988). Maternal narcotic abuse and the newborn. *Archives of Diseases in Childhood* 63(1): 81–3.

Armant, D.R., Saunders, D.E. (1996). Exposure of embryonic cells to alcohol: contrasting effects during preimplantation development. *Seminars in Perinatology* 20(2): 127–39.

Ballard, J.L, Khoury, J.C., Wedig, K., Wang, L., Eilers-Walsman, B.L., Lipp, R. (1991). New Ballard Score, expanded to include extremely premature infants. *Journal of Pediatrics* 119(3): 417–23.

Banks, M. (2001). Breech birth beyond the 'term breech trial'. *Birthspirit Midwifery Journal*. Available at http://www.birthspirit.co.nz/Articles/Articles/Breech%20birth%20beyond%20 the%20TBT.pdf (accessed 1 October 2009).

Bardy, A.H., Seppälä, T., Lillsunde, P., Kataja, J.M., Koskela, P., Pikkarainen, J., Hiilesmaa, V.K. (1993). Objectively measured tobacco exposure during pregnancy: neonatal effects and relation to maternal smoking. *British Journal of Obstetrics and Gynaecology* 100(8): 721–6.

Barnes, N. (2007). Preconceptual care: why we need foresight. Part 2: from pollution to pesticides. *Practising Midwife* 10(11): 34–5.

Baston, H., Durward, H. (2001). *Examination of the newborn: a practical guide*. London, Routledge.

Baxley, E., Gobbo, R. (2004). Shoulder dystocia. *American Family Physician* 69(7): 1707.

BBC. (2006). *Spanish woman is oldest mother*. Available at http://news.bbc.co.uk/1/hi/ health/6220523.stm (accessed 3 October 2009).

BBC. (2009). *World's oldest mother dies aged 69*. Available at http://news.bbc.co.uk/1/hi/ health/8152002.stm (accessed 3 October 2009).

Beal, S.M., Byard, R.W. (1995). Accidental death or sudden infant death syndrome? *Journal of Paediatrics and Child Health* 31(4): 269–71.

Berbey, R., Manduley, A., Vigil-De Gracia, P. (2001). Counting fetal movements as a universal test for fetal wellbeing. *International Journal of Gynecology and Obstetrics* 74(3): 293–5.

Best, J. (2007). Rubella. *Seminars in Fetal and Neonatal Medicine* 12(3): 182–92.

Boivin, J.F. (1997). Risk of spontaneous abortion in women occupationally exposed to anaesthetic gases: a meta-analysis. *Occupational Environmental Medicine* 54(8): 541–8.

Bowlby, J. (1953). *Child care and the growth of love*. London, Penguin.

British Medical Association and Royal Pharmaceutical Society of Great Britain. (2008). *British National Formulary*. London, BMJ Group and RPS Publishing.

Campbell, M.K. (1998). Factors affecting outcome in post-term birth. *Current Opinion in Obstetrics and Gynaecology* 9(6): 356–60.

Campion, P., Owen, L., McNeill, A., McGuire, C. (1994). Evaluation of a mass media campaign on smoking and pregnancy. *Addiction* 89(10): 1245–54.

Capstick, B. (ed.) (1993). *Litigation: a risk management guide for midwives*. London: Royal College of Midwives.

Caughey, A., Stotland, N., Washington, A.E., Escobar, G.J. (2009). Who is at risk for prolonged and postterm pregnancy? *American Journal of Obstetrics and Gynecology* 200(6): 683.e1–5. Epub 2009 Apr 19.

Chan, A., McCaul, K.A., Cundy, P.J., Haan, E.A., Byron-Scott, R. (1997). Perinatal risk factors for developmental dysplasia of the hip. *Archives of Disease in Childhood* 76(2): F94–100.

Chaplin, J., McDiarmid, P. (1992). Teenage parenthood – myth and reality. *Community Health Action* 25(Autumn): 3.

Chen, X., Wen, S., Fleming, N., Demissie, K., Rhoads, G.G., Walker, M. (2007). Teenage pregnancy and adverse birth outcomes: a large population based retrospective cohort study. *International Journal of Epidemiology* 36(2): 368–73.

Cheng, P., Shaw, S., Yoong, Y. (2006). Association of fetal choroid plexus cysts with trisomy 18 in a population previously screened by nuchal translucency thickness measurement. *Journal of the Society for Gynecologic Investigation* 13(4): 280–4.

Christopher, E. (1996). Family planning and reproductive decision making. In C. Niven, A. Walker (eds). *Reproductive potential and fertility control*. Oxford, Butterworth Heinemann.

Cicero, S., Spencer, K., Avgidou, K., Faiola, S., Nicolaides, K.H. (2005). Maternal serum biochemistry at 11–13+6 weeks in relation to the presence or absence of the fetal nasal bone on ultrasonography in chromosomally abnormal fetuses: an updated analysis of integrated ultrasound and biochemical screening. *Prenatal Diagnosis* 25(11): 977–83.

Cleary-Goldman, J., Malone, F., Vidaver, J. (2005). Impact of maternal age on obstetric outcome. *Obstetrics and Gynecology* 105(5): 983–90.

Cluett, E.R., Burns, E. (2008). Immersion in water in labour and birth. *Cochrane Database of Systematic Reviews* 4: CD000111.

Cnattingius, S., Haglund, B. (1997). Decreasing smoking prevalence during pregnancy in Sweden: the effect on small for gestational age births. *American Journal of Public Health* 87(3): 410–13.

Coates, T. (2003). *Malpositions of the occiput and malpresentations: Myles textbook for midwives*. Edinburgh, Churchill Livingstone.

Cohen-Overbeek, T., Grijseels, E., Niemeijer, N., Hop, W.C., Wladimiroff, J.W., Tibboel, D. (2008). Isolated or non-isolated duodenal obstruction: perinatal outcome following prenatal or postnatal diagnosis. *Ultrasound in Obstetrics and Gynecology* 32(6): 784–92.

Crompton, J. (1996). Post-traumatic stress disorder and childbirth. *British Journal of Midwifery* 4(6): 290–5.

Dare, M.R., Middleton, P., Crowther, C.A., Flenady, V., Varatharaju, B. (2006). Planned early birth versus expectant management (waiting) for prelabour rupture of membranes at term (37 weeks or more). *Cochrane Database of Systematic Reviews* 1: CD005302.

Denner, S. (1995). Extending professional practice: benefits and pitfalls. *Nursing Times* 91(14): 27–9.

Department of Health. (1993a). *Changing childbirth*. London, HMSO.

Department of Health. (1993b) *Clinical audit: meeting and improving standards in health care*. Heywood, UK, Health Publications Unit.

Department of Health. (1997). *The new NHS: modern, dependable*. London, Department of Health.

Department of Health. (2004). *National service framework for children, young people and maternity services*. Standard 11. Maternity Services. London, Department of Health.

Department of Health. (2005). *Mental capacity act*. London, HMSO.

Department of Health. (2007). *Maternity matters: choice, access and continuity of care in a safe service*. London, Department of Health.

Department of Health. (2008). *The child health programme: pregnancy and the first five years of life*. London, Department for Children, Schools and Families.

Department of Health. (2009a). *Local data on pregnant women smoking at time of delivery*. Available at http://www.dh.gov.uk/en/Publichealth/Healthimprovement/Tobacco/Tobaccogeneralinformation/DH_4139682 (accessed 11 October 2009).

Department of Health. (2009b). *Reference guide to consent for examination or treatment*, 2nd edn. London, Department of Health. Available at http://www.dh.gov.uk/prod_consum_dh/groups/dh_digitalassets/documents/digitalasset/dh_103653.pdf (accessed 26 September 2009).

Department of Health. (2009c). *Reduce the risk of cot death*. Available at http://www.dh.gov.uk/dr_consum_dh/groups/dh_digitalassets/documents/digitalasset/dh_096299.pdf (accessed 9 October 2009).

Deshpande, S.A., Jog, S., Watson, H., Gornall, A. (2009). Do babies with isolated single umbilical artery need routine postnatal renal ultrasonography? *Archives of Disease in Childhood Fetal and Neonatal Edition* 94(4): F265–7.

Dezateux, C., Rosendahl, K. (2007). Developmental dysplasia of the hip. *Lancet* 369(9572): 1541–52.

Dimond, B. (2006). *Legal aspects of midwifery*, 3rd edn. Edinburgh, Butterworth Heinemann.

Doggett, C., Burrett, S.L., Osborn, D. (2005). Home visits during pregnancy and after birth for women with an alcohol or drug problem. *Cochrane Database of Systematic Reviews* 4: CD004456.

Donabedian, A. (1966). Evaluating the quality of medical care. *Millbank Memorial Fund* 44(3 Suppl): 166–206.

Dowling, S., Martin, R., Skidmore, P., Doyal, L., Cameron, A., Lloyd, S. (1996). Nurses taking on junior doctors' work: a confusion of accountability. *BMJ* 312(7040): 1211–14.

English, D.R., Hulse, G.K., Milne, E., Holman, C.D., Bower, C.I. (1997). Maternal cannabis use and low birth weight: a meta-analysis. *Addiction* 92(11): 1553–60

Enkin, M.W., Keirse, M.J.N.C., Renfrew, M.J., Neilson, J.P. (eds). (1995). *Pregnancy and childbirth module of the Cochrane Database of Systematic Reviews*. London, MJ Publishing.

Faiola, S., Tsoi, E., Huggon, I., Allan, L.D., Nicolaides, K.H. (2005). Likelihood ratio for trisomy 21 in fetuses with tricuspid regurgitation at the 11 to 13+6-week scan. *Ultrasound in Obstetrics and Gynecology* 26(1): 22–7.

Falcon, O., Auer, M., Gerovassili, A., Spencer, K., Nicolaides, K.H. (2006). Screening for trisomy 21 by fetal tricuspid regurgitation, nuchal translucency and maternal serum free beta-hCG and PAPP-A at 11 + 0 to 13 + 6 weeks. *Ultrasound in Obstetrics and Gynecology* 27(2): 151–5.

Food Standards Agency. (2008). *Eat well, be well, alcohol*. Available at www.eatwell.gov.uk/healthydiet/nutritionessentials/drinks/alcohol/ (accessed 3 October 2009).

Franko, K., Gluckman, P., Law, C., Beedle, A., Morton, S., Kiess, W., Chernausek, S.D., Hokken-Koelega, A.C.S. (eds). (2008). Low birth weight and optimal fetal development: a global perspective. In W. Kiess, S.D. Chernaussek, A.C.S. Hokken-Koelega (eds). *Small for gestational age: causes and consequences*. Basel, Karger.

Freeborn, S.F., Calvert, R.T., Black, P., Macfarlane, T., D'Souza, S.W. (1980). Saliva and blood pethidine concentrations in the mother and newborn baby. *British Journal of Obstetrics and Gynaecology* 87(11): 966–9.

Friedberg, M., Silverman, N., Moon-Grady, A., Tong, E., Nourse, J., Sorenson, B., Lee, J., Hornberger, L.K. (2009). Prenatal detection of congenital heart disease. *Journal of Pediatrics* 155(1): 26–31.

Gamsu, H. (1993). The effects of pain relief on the baby. In G. Chamberlain, A. Wraight, P. Steer (eds). *Pain and its relief in childbirth*. Edinburgh, Churchill Livingstone.

Geary, M., Crowley, D., Boylan, P. (1997). Passive cigarette smoking in pregnancy. *Journal of Obstetrics and Gynaecology* 17(3): 264–5.

General Medical Council. (2006). *Good medical practice*. Available at http://www.gmc-uk. org/guidance/good_medical_practice/good_clinical_care/index.asp (accessed 13 September 2009).

Gerscovich, E.O. (1997). A radiologist's guide to the imaging in the diagnosis and treatment of developmental dysplasia of the hip. General considerations, physical examination as applied to real-time sonography and radiography. *Skeletal Radiology* 26(7): 386–97.

Gillies, P., Wakefield, M. (1993). Smoking in pregnancy. *Current Obstetrics and Gynaecology* 3(3): 157–61.

Goffinet, F., Carayol M., Foidart, J., Alexander, S., Uzan, S., Subtil, D., Bréart, G.; PREMODA Study Group. (2006). Is planned vaginal delivery for breech presentation at term still an option? Results of an observational prospective survey in France and Belgium. *American Journal of Obstetrics and Gynecology* 194(4): 1002–11.

Goodwin, R., Canino, G., Ortega, A., Bird, H.R. (2009). Maternal mental health and childhood asthma among Puerto Rican youth: the role of prenatal smoking. *Journal of Asthma* 46(7): 726–30.

Green, J., Statham, H. (1993). Testing for abnormality in routine antenatal care. *Midwifery* 9(3): 124–35.

Green, J., Kitzinger, J., Coupland, V.A. (1990). Stereotypes of childbearing women: a look at some evidence. *Midwifery* 6(4): 125–32.

Green, J., Hewison, J., Bekker, H., Bryant, L.D., Cuckle, H.S. (2004). Psychosocial aspects of genetic screening for pregnant women and newborns: a systematic review. *Health Technology Assessment* 8(33).

Greig, C. (2003). Trauma during birth: haemorrhage and convulsions. In D.M. Fraser, M.A. Cooper (eds). *Myles textbook for midwives*. Edinburgh, Churchill Livingstone.

Gülmezoglu, A.M., Crowther, C.A., Middleton, P. (2006). Induction of labour for improving birth outcomes for women at or beyond term. *Cochrane Database of Systematic Reviews* 4: CD004945.

Gupta, J., Cave, M., Lilford, R., Farrell, T.A., Irving, H.C., Mason, G., Hau, C.M. (1995). Clinical significance of fetal choroid plexus cysts. *Lancet* 346(8977): 724–9.

Håberg, S., Bentdal, Y., London, S., Kvaerner, K.J., Nystad, W., Nafstad, P. (2010). Prenatal and postnatal parental smoking and acute otitis media in early childhood. *Acta Paediatrica* 99(1): 99–105.

Haglund, B., Cnattingius, S. (1990). Cigarette smoking as a risk factor for sudden infant death syndrome, a population based study. *American Journal of Public Health* 80(1): 29–32.

Hall, D.M.B. (1996). *Health for all children*. Oxford, Oxford University Press.

Hall, D.M.B. (1999). The role of the routine neonatal examination (Editorial). *British Medical Journal* 318(7184): 19–20.

Hall, D., Elliman, D. (2006). *Health for all children*, 4th edn. Oxford, Oxford University Press.

Hall, M.H., Chng, P.K., Macgillivray, I. (1980). Is antenatal care worthwhile. *Lancet* 2(8185): 78–80.

Hampshire, S. (1984). *The maternal instinct*. Glasgow, Collins.

Hannah, M., Hodnett, E., Willan, A.R., Foster, G.A., Di Cecco, R., Helewa, M. (2000a). Prelabour rupture of the membranes at term: expectant management at home or in hospital? The Term PROM study Group. *Obstetrics and Gynecology* 96(4): 533–8.

Hannah, M.E., Hannah, W., Hewson, S.A. Hodnett, E.D., Saigal, S., Willan, A.R. (2000b). Planned caesarean section versus planned vaginal birth for breech presentation at term: a randomised multicentre trial. *Lancet* 356(9239): 1375–83.

Haugland, S., Haug, K. and Wold, B. (1996). The pregnant smoker's experience of ante-natal care – results from a qualitative study. *Scandinavian Journal of Primary Health Care* 14(4): 216–22.

Haverkamp, A.D., Orleans, M., Langenoerfer, S., McFee, J., Murphy, J. (1979). A controlled trial of the different effects of intrapartum fetal monitoring. *American Journal of Obstetrics and Gynaecology* 134(4): 399–412.

Hawkins, S., Cole, T., Law, C. (2009). Examining the relationship between maternal employment and health behaviours in 5 year old British children. *Journal of Epidemiology and Community Health*. Available at http://dx.doi.org/10.1136/jech.2008.084590 (accessed 11 October 2009).

Haworth, S.G., Bull, C. (1993). Physiology of congenital heart disease. *Archives of Disease in Childhood* 68(5): 707–11.

Hayes, J., Dave, S., Rogers, C., Quist-Therson, E., Townsend, J. (2003). A national survey in England of the routine examination of the newborn baby. *Midwifery* 19(4): 277–84.

Hecht, S.S. (2003). Tobacco carcinogens, their biomarkers and tobacco-induced cancer. *Nature Reviews Cancer* 3(10): 733–44.

Herbst, A., Kallen, K. (2007). Time between membrane rupture and delivery and septicemia in term neonates. *Obstetrics and Gynecology* 110(3): 612–18.

Hilder, L., Costeloe, K., Thiganathan, B. (1998). Prolonged pregnancy: evaluating gestation specific risks of fetal and infant mortality. *British Journal of Obstetrics and Gynaecology* 105(2): 169–73.

Hilton, T. (1991). *The Great Ormond Street book of baby and child care*. London, BCA.

Honeyfield, M. (2009). Neonatal nurse practitioners: past, present, and future. *Advances in Neonatal Care* 9(3): 91–2.

Hu, H., Téllez-Rojo, M., Bellinger, D., Smith, D., Ettinger, A.S., Lamadrid-Figueroa, H., Schwartz, J., Schnaas, L., Mercado-García, A., Hernández-Avila, M. (2006). Fetal lead exposure at each stage of pregnancy as a predictor of infant mental development. *Environmental Health Perspectives* 114(11): 1730–5.

Huizink, A., Bartels, M., Rose, R., Pulkkinen, L., Eriksson, C.J., Kaprio, J. (2008). Chernobyl exposure as stressor during pregnancy and hormone levels in adolescent offspring. *Journal of Epidemiol Community Health* 62(4): e5.

Hull, D., Johnston, D.I. (1993). *Essential paediatrics*, 3rd edn. Edinburgh, Churchill Livingstone.

Human Fertilisation and Embryology Authority. (2009). Funding and payment issues: NHS fertility treatment. http://www.hfea.gov.uk/fertility.html (accessed 3 October 2009).

Hutcherson, A. (2010). Critical relection on a midwife's development and practice in relation to examination of the newborn. *Midwives* (December/January): 1–9.

Jacob, J., Pfenninger, J. (1997). Cesarean deliveries: when is a paediatrician necessary? *Obstetrics and Gynaecology* 89(2): 217–20.

Jennings, S.E. (ed.) (1995). *Infertility counselling*. Oxford, Blackwell Science.

Jensen, T.K., Hjollund, N.H.I., Henriksen, T.B., Scheike, T., Kolstad, H., Giwercman, A., Ernst, E., Bonde, J.P., Skakkebaek, N.E., Olsen, J. (1998). Does moderate alcohol consumption affect fertility? Follow-up study among couples planning first pregnancy. *British Medical Journal* 317(7157): 505–10.

Johanson, R., Menon, V. (1999). Vacuum extraction versus forceps for assisted vaginal delivery. *Cochrane Database of Systematic Reviews* 2: CD000224.

Johnson, J., Aldrich, M., Angelus, P., Stevenson, D.K., Smith, D.W., Herschel, M.J., Papagaroufalis, C., Valaes, T. (1984). Oxytocin and neonatal hyperbilirubinaemia: studies of bilirubin production. *American Journal of Diseases in Childhood* 138(11): 1047–50.

Jones, K.L. (1997). *Smith's recognizable patterns of human malformation*. Philadelphia: W.B. Saunders Company.

Jones, K.L., Smith, D.W. (1973). Recognition of fetal alcohol syndrome in infancy. *Lancet* 302(7836): 999–1001.

Jong, E., De Haan, T., Kroesb, A., Beersma, M.F.C., Oepkes, D., Walther, F.J. (2006). Parvovirus B19 infection in pregnancy. *Journal of Clinical Virology* 36(1): 1–7.

Jorgensen, F.S. (1995). User acceptability of an alpha feto-protein screening programme. *Danish Medical Bulletin* 42(1): 100–5.

Kagan, K., Cicero, S., Staboulidou, I., Wright, D., Nicolaides, K.H. (2009). Fetal nasal bone in screening for trisomies 21, 18 and 13 and Turner syndrome at 11–13 weeks of gestation. *Ultrasound in Obstetrics and Gynecology* 33(3): 259–64.

Katalinic, A., Rösch, C., Ludwig, M., German ICSI Follow-Up Study Group. (2004). Pregnancy course and outcome after intracytoplasmic sperm injection: a controlled, prospective cohort study. *Fertility and Sterility* 81(6): 1604–16.

Kaufman, M.H. (1997). The teratogenic affects of alcohol exposure during pregnancy, and its influence on the chromosome constitution of the pre-ovulatory egg. *Alcohol and Alcoholism* 32(2): 113–28.

Kelso, I.M., Parsons, R.J., Lawrence, G.F., Arora, S.S., Edmonds, D.K., Cooke, I.D. (1978). An assessment of continuous fetal heart rate monitoring in labour: a randomised trial. *American Journal of Obstetrics and Gynaecology* 131(5): 526–32.

Keren, R., Bhutani, V., Luan, X., Nihtianova, S., Cnaan, A., Schwartz, J. (2005). Identifying newborns at risk of significant hyperbilirubinaemia: a comparison of two recommended approaches. *Archives of Disease in Childhood* 90(4): 415–21.

Kesmodel, U., Wisborg, K., Olsen, S.F. Henriksen, T.B., Secher, N.J. (2002). Moderate alcohol intake during pregnancy and the risk of still birth and death in the first year of life. *American Journal of Epidemiology* 155(4): 305–12.

Knowles, R., Griebsch, I., Dezateux, C., Brown, J., Bull, C., Wren, C. (2005). Newborn screening for congenital heart defects: a systematic review and cost-effectiveness analysis. *Health Technology Assessment* 9(44).

Kumar, V., Abbas, A., Fausto, N. (2004). *Robbins and Cotran's pathologic basis of disease*, 7th edn. Edinburgh, Elsevier.

Ladfors, L., Mattsson, L.A., Eriksson, M., Fall, O. (1996). A randomised trial of two expectant managements of prelabour rupture of the membranes at 34 to 42 weeks. *British Journal of Obstetrics and Gynaecology* 103(8): 755–62.

Leigh, B., Milgrom, J. (2008). Risk factors for antenatal depression, postnatal depression and parenting stress. *BMC Psychiatry* 8(24). Available at http://www.biomedcentral.com/bmcpsychiatry/ (accessed 6 October 2009).

Leonard, M., Graham, S., Bonacum, D. (2004). The human factor: the critical importance of effective teamwork and communication in providing safe care. *Quality and Safety in Health Care* 13(Suppl.1): i85–90.

Li, P., McLaughlin J., Infante-Rivard, C. (2009). Maternal occupational exposure to extremely low frequency magnetic fields and the risk of brain cancer in the offspring. *Cancer Causes and Control* 20(6): 945–55.

Liao, C., Wei, J., Li, Q., Li, L., Li, J., Li, D. (2006). Efficacy and safety of cordocentesis for prenatal diagnosis. *International Journal of Gynecology and Obstetrics* 93(1): 13–17.

Lieberman, E., O'Donoghue, C. (2002). Unintended effects of epidural analgesia during labour: a systematic review. *American Journal of Obstetrics and Gynecology* 186(5 Suppl.): s31–68.

Lieberman, E., Lang, J., Frigoletto, F., Richardson, D.K., Ringer, S.A., Cohen, A. (1997). Epidural analgesia, intrapartum fever, and neonatal sepsis evaluation. *Pediatrics* 99(3): 415–19.

Lindsay, P. (2004). Bleeding in pregnancy. In C. Henderson, S. Macdonald (eds). *Mayes' midwifery: a textbook for midwives*, 13th edn. Edinburgh, Balliere Tindall.

Lissauer, T.J., Steer, P. (1986). The relation between the need for intubation at birth, abnormal cardiotocograms in labour and cord artery blood gas and pH values. *British Journal of Obstetrics and Gynaecology* 93(10): 1060–6.

Lopez, J., Reich, D. (2006). Choroid plexus cysts. *Journal of the American Board of Family Medicine* 19(4): 422–5.

Lowry, C., Donovan, V., Murphy, J. (2005). Auditing hip ultrasound screening of infants at increased risk of developmental dysplasia of the hip. *Archives of Disease in Childhood* 90(6): 579–81.

Lumley, J., Chamberlain, C., Dowswell, T., Oliver, S., Oakley, L., Watson, L. (2008). Interventions for promoting smoking cessation during pregnancy. *Cochrane Database of Systematic Reviews* 4: CD001055.

Lumsden, H. (2002). Physical assessment of the newborn: a holistic approach. *British Journal of Midwifery* 10(4): 205–9.

McCarthy, F., Jones, C., Rowlands, S., Giles, M. (2009). Primary and secondary cytomegalovirus in pregnancy. *Obstetrician and Gynaecologist* 11(2): 96–100.

MacDonald, D., Grant, A., Sheridan-Pereira, M., Boylan, P., Chalmers, I. (1985). The Dublin randomised controlled trial of intrapartum fetal heart rate monitoring. *American Journal of Obstetrics and Gynaecology* 152(5): 524–39.

McDonald, S. (2008). Examining a newborn baby: are midwives using their skills? *British Journal of Midwifery* 16(11): 722–4.

McFarlane, J., Parker, B., Soeken, K. (1996). Physical abuse, smoking, and substance use during pregnancy: prevalence, interrelationships, and effects on birth weight. *Journal of Obstetric, Gynaecological and Neonatal Nursing* 25(4): 313–20.

McIver, L. (2007). Substance misuse: what's the problem? In G. Edwards, S. Byrom (eds). *Essential midwifery practice: public health*. Oxford, Blackwell Publishing.

MacKeith, N. (1995). Who should examine the normal neonate. *Nursing Times* 91(14): 34–5.

McKenna, A., Woolwich, C., Burgess, K. (1994). The emergency nurse practitioner. In L. Sbaih (ed.). *Issues in accident and emergency nursing*. London, Chapman & Hall.

McNamara, J. (1995). *Bruised before birth: parenting children exposed to parental substance abuse*. London, British Agencies for Adoption and Fostering.

McNamara, S., Giguère, V., St-Louis, L., Boileau, J. (2009). Development and implementation of the specialized nurse practitioner role: use of the PEPPA framework to achieve success. *Nursing and Health Sciences* 11(3): 318–25.

Mahan, S., Katz, J., Kim, Y. (2009). To screen or not to screen? A decision analysis of the utility of screening for developmental dysplasia of the hip. *Journal of Bone and Joint Surgery (American)* 91(7): 1705–19.

Mahle, W., Newburger, J., Matherne, G., Smith, F.C., Hoke, T.R., Koppel, R., Gidding, S.S., Beekman, R.H., 3rd, Grosse, S.D. (2009). Role of pulse oximetry in examining newborns for congenital heart disease: a scientific statement from the AHA and AAP. *Pediatrics* 124(2): 823–36.

Makrydimas, G., Sotiriadis, A., Huggon, I., *et al.* (2005). Nuchal translucency and fetal cardiac defects: a pooled analysis of major fetal echocardiography centers. *American Journal of Obstetrics and Gynecology* 192(1): 89–95.

Malpas, T., Darlow, B. (1999). Neonatal abstinence syndrome following abrupt cessation of breastfeeding. *New Zealand Medical Journal* 112(1080): 12–13.

Martin, R. (1997). Changing boundaries and legal risk: a challenge for nursing. *Health Care Risk Report* June: 13–15.

Mattingly, J.E., D'Alessio, J., Ramanathan, J. (2003). Effects of obstetric analgesics and anesthetics on the neonate: a review. *Paediatric Drugs* 5(9): 615–27.

Medical Research Council. (1991). Prevention of neural tube defects: results of the Medical Research Council Vitamin Study. MRC Vitamin Study Group. *Lancet* 338(8760): 131–7.

Mercier, F.J., Benhamou, D. (1997). Hyperthermia related to epidural analgesia during labor. *International Journal of Obstetric Anaesthesia* 6(1): 19–24.

Michaelides, S. (1995). A deeper knowledge. *Nursing Times* 91(35): 59–61.

Michaelides, S. (1997). Newborn examination: whose responsibility? *British Journal of Midwifery* 5(9): 538.

Mitchell, M. (2003). Midwives conducting the neonatal examination: part 1. *British Journal of Midwifery* 11(1): 16–21.

Mollberg, M., Hagberg, H., Bager, B., Lilja, H., Ladfors, L. (2005). High birth weight and shoulder dystocia: the strongest risk factors for obstetrical brachial plexus palsy in a Swedish population-based study. *Acta Obstetricia et Gynecologica Scandinavica* 84(7): 654–9.

Montoya, J., Remington, J. (2008). Management of *Toxoplasma gondii* infection during pregnancy. *Clinical Practice* 47(4): 554–66.

Myhra, W., Davis, M., Mueller, B.A., Hickok, D. (1992). Maternal smoking and the risk of polyhydramnios. *American Journal of Public Health* 82(2): 176–9.

Mylonakis, E., Paliou, M., Hohmann, E., Calderwood, S.B., Wing, E.J. (2002). Listeriosis during pregnancy: a case series and review of 222 cases. *Medicine (Baltimore)* 81(4): 260–9.

National Institute for Health and Clinical Excellence. (2004). *Fertility: assessment and treatment for people with fertility problems*. London, NICE. Available at http://www.rcog.org.uk/files/rcog-corp/uploaded-files/NEBFertilityFull.pdf (accessed 3 October 2009).

National Institute for Health and Clinical Excellence. (2006). *Routine postnatal care of women and their babies*. London, NICE.

National Institute for Health and Clinical Excellence. (2007). *Intrapartum care: care of healthy women and their babies during childbirth*. NICE clinical guideline 55. London, NICE.

National Institute for Health and Clinical Excellence. (2008). *Antenatal care: routine care for the healthy pregnant woman*. NICE clinical guideline 62. London, NICE.

National Statistics. (2009). *Fertility*. Available at http://www.statistics.gov.uk/cci/nugget.asp?ID=951 (accessed 3 October 2009).

Nesbitt, T.S., Gilbert, W.M., Herrchen, B. (1999). Shoulder dystocia and associated risk factors with macrosomic infants born in California. *American Journal of Obstetrics and Gynecology* 180(4): 1047.

Neuspiel, D.R., Rush, D., Butler, N.R., Golding, J., Bijur, P.E., Kurzon, M. (1989). Parental smoking and post-infancy wheezing in children: a prospective cohort study. *American Journal of Public Health* 79(2): 168–71.

NHS Quality Improvement Scotland. (2004). *Best practice statement – May 2004: routine examination of the newborn*. Available at http://www.nhshealthquality.org/nhsqis/files/20219%20BPS_Newborn%20.pdf (accessed 11 October 2009).

NHS Quality Improvement Scotland. (2008). *Best practice statement – May 2008: routine Examination of the newborn*. Available at http://www.nhshealthquality.org/nhsqis/files/Routine%20Examination%20of%20the%20Newborn%20BPS%202008.pdf (accessed 11 October 2009).

Nora, J.G. (1990). Perinatal cocaine use: maternal, fetal and neonatal effects. *Neonatal Network* 9(2): 45–52.

Nursing and Midwifery Council. (2004). *Midwives rules and standards*. London, NMC.

Nursing and Midwifery Council. (2008a). *The code: standards of conduct, performance and ethics for nurses and midwives*. London, NMC.

Nursing and Midwifery Council. (2008b). *The Prep handbook*. London, NMC.

Nursing and Midwifery Council. (2009). *Record keeping: guidance for nurses and midwives*. London, NMC.

Oddie, S., Embleton, N.D. (2002). Risk factors for early onset neonatal group B streptococcal sepsis: case–control study. *BMJ* 325(7359): 308.

Odent, M. (1998). Use of water during labour – updated recommendations. *MIDIRS Midwifery Digest* 8(1): 68–9.

Office for National Statistics and Teenage Pregnancy Unit. (2009). *Under 18 and under 16 conception rates*. Available at http://www.dcsf.gov.uk/everychildmatters/resources-and-practice/IG00200/ (accessed 2 October 2009).

Okti-Poki, H., Holland, A., Pitkin, J. (2005). Double bubble, double trouble. *Pediatric Surgery International* 21(6): 428–31.

Olesen, A.W., Westergaard, J.G., Olsen, J. (2003). Perinatal and maternal complications related to postterm delivery: a national register-based study, 1978–1993. *American Journal of Obstetrics and Gynecology* 189(1): 222–7.

Olofsson, C.H., Ekblom, A., Ekman-Ordeberg, G., Hjelm, A., Irested, L. (1996). Lack of analgesic effect of systematically administered morphine or pethidine on labour pain. *British Journal of Obstetrics and Gynaecology* 103(10): 968–72.

Pairman, S., Pincombe, J., Thorogood, C., Tracy, S. (2006). *Midwifery – preparing for practice*. Marickville, Elsevier-Australia.

Piper, J.M., Newton, E.R., Berkus, M.D., Peairs, W.A. (1998). Meconium: a marker for peripartum infection. *Obstetrics and Gynaecology* 91(5): 741–5.

Plessinger, M.A. (1998). Prenatal exposure to amphetamines: risks and adverse outcomes in pregnancy. *Obstetrics and Gynaecology Clinics of North America* 25(1): 119–38.

Polin, R.A., Fox, W.W. (1998). *Fetal and neonatal physiology*, vol. 1, 2nd edn. Philadelphia, WB Saunders Company.

Prochaska, J.O., DiClemente, C.C. (1983). Stages and processes of self-change of smoking: towards an integrative model. *Journal of Consulting and Clinical Psychology* 51(3): 390–5.

Quinlivan, J. (2004). Teenagers who plan parenthood. *Sexual Health* 1(4): 201–8.

Ramsay, C.R., Glazener, C.M.A., Campbell, M.K., Booth, P., Duffty, P., Lloyd, D.J., McDonald, A., Reid, J.A. (1997). Neonatal screening examinations: is one examination enough? *Journal of Epidemiology and Community Health* 51(5): 606.

Raphael-Leff, J. (1991). *Psychological processes of childbearing*. London, Chapman & Hall.

Redshaw, M., Rowe, R., Hockley, C., Brocklehurst, P. (2007). *Recorded delivery: a national survey of women's experience of maternity care*. Oxford, National Perinatal Epidemiology Unit.

Richardson, G.A., Goldschmidt, L., Larkby, C. (2007). Effects of prenatal cocaine exposure on growth: a longitudinal analysis. *Pediatrics* 120(4): 1017–27.

Richmond, S., Reay, G., Abu Harb, M. (2002). Routine pulse oximetry in the asymptomatic newborn. *Archives of Disease in Childhood Fetal and Neonatal Edition* 87(2): 83–8.

Richter, L., Norris, S., Ginsburg, C. (2006). The silent truth of teenage pregnancies – Birth to Twenty cohort's next generation. *South African Medical Journal* 96(2): 122–3.

Roach, V.J., Rogers, M.S. (1997). Pregnancy outcome beyond 41 weeks gestation. *International Journal of Gynaecology and Obstetrics* 59(1): 19–24.

Roberton, N.R.C. (1996). *A manual of normal neonatal care*, 2nd edn. London, Arnold.

Robinson, J.S., Moore, V.M., Owens, J.A., McMillen, I.C. (2000). Origins of fetal growth restriction. *European Journal of Obstetrics, Gynecology, and Reproductive Biology* 92(1): 13–19.

Roch, S., Alexander, J., Levey, V. (1990). *Postnatal care: a research-based approach*. London, Macmillan.

Rogers, J. (1997). It could be you: antenatal screening. *Nursing Times* 93(6): 54–5.

Romundstad, L., Romundstad, P., Sunde, A., von Düring, V., Skjaerven, R., Gunnell, D., Vatten, L.J. (2008). Effects of technology or maternal factors on perinatal outcome after assisted fertilisation: a population-based cohort study. *Lancet* 372(9640): 737–43.

Rothman, B.K. (1988). *The tentative pregnancy prenatal diagnosis and the future of motherhood*. London, Pandora.

Royal College of Nursing. (2002). *Clinical supervision in the workplace: guidance for occupational health nurses*. Available at http://www.rcn.org.uk/__data/assets/pdf_file/0007/78523/001549. pdf (accessed 25 September 2009).

Royal College of Obstetricians and Gynaecologists. (2002). *The investigation and management of the small-for-gestational age fetus*. RCOG Green Top Guideline No. 31. Available at http://www.rcog.org.uk/files/rcog-corp/uploaded-files/GT31SmallGestationalAgeFetus.pdf (accessed 28 February 2010).

Royal College of Obstetricians and Gynaecologists. (2005). *Operative vaginal delivery*. Guideline No. 26. London, RCOG. Available at http://www.rcog.org.uk/files/rcog-corp/uploaded-files/GT26OperativeVaginalDelivery2005.pdf (accessed 2 October 2009).

Royal College of Obstetricians and Gynaecologists. (2006a). *Alcohol consumption and the outcomes of pregnancy*. Statement No. 5. London, RCOG. Available at http://www.rcog.org.uk/files/rcog-corp/uploaded-files/RCOGStatement5AlcoholPregnancy2006.pdf (accessed 28 February 2010).

Royal College of Obstetricians and Gynaecologists. (2006b). *RCOG Green Top Guidelines: the management of breech presentation*. Guideline No. 20b. London, RCOG.

Salvesen, K.A., Eik-nes, S.H. (1999). Ultrasound during pregnancy and subsequent childhood non-right handedness: a meta-analysis. *Ultrasound in Obstetrics and Gynaecology* 13(4): 241–6.

Salvesen, K.A., Bakketeig, L.S., Eik-nes, S.H., Undheim, J.O., Okland, O. (1992). Routine ultrasonography *in utero* and school performance at age 8–9 years. *Lancet* 339(8785): 85–9.

Saraf, S. (2009). Facial laceration at caesarean section: experience with tissue adhesive. *Eplasty* 9: e3. Epub 2009 Jan 9.

Sarker, P., Hill, L. (1996). Maternal anxiety and depression – the experience of prolonged pregnancy. *Journal of Obstetrics and Gynaecology* 16(6): 488–92.

Sauerbrei, A., Wutzler, P. (2007). Herpes simplex and varicella-zoster virus infections during pregnancy: current concepts of prevention, diagnosis and therapy. Part 2: varicella-zoster virus infections. *Medical Microbiology and Immunology* 196(2): 95–102.

Savrin, C. (2009). Growth and development of the nurse practitioner role around the globe. *Journal of Pediatric Health Care* 23(5): 310–14.

Schellscheidt, J., Øyen, N., Jorch, G. (1997). Interactions between maternal smoking and other prenatal risk factors for sudden infant death syndrome (SIDS). *Acta Paediatrica* 86(8): 857–63.

Seidel, H.M., Rosenstein, B.J., Pathak, A. (1997). *Primary care of the newborn*, 2nd edn. London, Mosby.

Shea, K.M., Wilcox, A.J., Little, R.E. (1998). Postterm delivery: a challenge for epidemiological research. *Epidemiology* 9(2): 199–204.

Shelton, K., Boivin, J. Hay, D, van den Bree, M.B.M., Rice, F.J., Harold, G.T., Thapar, A. (2009). Examining differences in psychological adjustment problems among children conceived by assisted reproductive technologies. *International Journal of Behavioural Development* 33(5): 385–92.

Shirangi, A., Fritschi L., Holman, C. (2008). Maternal occupational exposures and risk of spontaneous abortion in veterinary practice. *Journal of Occupational and Environmental Medicine* 65(11): 719–25.

Shirangi, A., Fritschi, L. Holman, C., Bower, C. (2009). Birth defects in offspring of female veterinarians. *Journal of Occupational and Environmental Medicine* 51(5): 525–33.

Simpson, C. (2004). Congenital abnormalities, fetal and neonatal surgery, and pain. In C. Henderson, S. Macdonald (eds). *Mayes' midwifery: a textbook for midwives*, 13th edn. Edinburgh, Balliere Tindall.

Smith, J.A., Mitchell, S. (1996). Debriefing after childbirth: a tool for effective risk management. *British Journal of Midwifery* 4(11): 581–6.

Smith, J.F., Hernandez, C., Wax, J.R. (1997). Fetal laceration injury at cesarean delivery. *Obstetrics and Gynaecology* 90(3): 344–6.

Smith, L., LaGasse, L., Derauf, C., Grant, P., Shah, R., Arria, A., Huestis, M., Haning, W., Strauss, A., Grotta, S.D., Jing, L., Lester, B.M. (2006). The Infant Development, Environment, and Lifestyle Study: effects of prenatal methamphetamine exposure, polydrug exposure, and poverty on intrauterine growth. *Pediatrics* 118(3): 1149–56.

Snijders, R., Noble, P., Sebire, N., Souka, A., Nicolaides, K.H. (1998). UK multicentre project on assessment of risk of trisomy 21 by maternal age and fetal nuchal translucency thickness at 10–14 weeks of gestation. *Lancet* 352(9125): 343–6.

Society of Obstetricians and Gynecologists of Canada. (2009). *SOGC clinical practice guideline, No. 226, June: vaginal delivery of breech presentation*. Available at http://www.sogc.org/guidelines/documents/gui226CPG0906.pdf (accessed 1 October 2009).

Sorahan, T., Hamilton, L., Gardiner, K., Hodgson, J.T., Harrington, J.M. (1999). Maternal occupational exposure to electromagnetic fields before, during and after pregnancy in relation to risks of childhood cancers: findings from the Oxford Survey of Childhood Cancers, 1953–1981 deaths. *American Journal of Industrial Medicine* 35(4): 348–57.

Statham, H., Green, J., Kafetsios, K. (1997). Who worries that something might be wrong with the baby? A prospective study of 1072 pregnant women. *Birth* 24(4): 223–33.

Steele, D. (2007). Examination of the newborn: why don't midwives use their skills. *British Journal of Midwifery* 15(12): 748–52.

Strachan, D.P., Cook, D.G. (1998). Health effects of passive smoking. 4. Parental smoking, middle ear disease and adenotonsillectomy in children. *Thorax* 53(1): 50–6.

Symon, A. (1997a). Midwives and litigation: allegations of clinical error. *British Journal of Midwifery* 5(1): 70–2.

Symon, A. (1997b). Recollections of staff: version of the truth. *British Journal of Midwifery* 15(7): 393–4.

Symon, A. (1998). Causation: a medico-legal problem. *British Journal of Midwifery* 6(3): 176–9.

The Information Centre. (2009). *NHS maternity statistics, England: 2007–2008*. Available at http://www.ic.nhs.uk/statistics-and-data-collections/hospital-care/maternity/nhs-maternity-statistics-england:-2007-08 (accessed 2 October 2009).

Thorpe-Raghdo, B. (1995). Newborn examinations – another delivery service. *MIDIRS Midwifery Digest* 5(4): 459.

Tolo, K.A., Little, R.E. (1993). Occasional binges by moderate drinkers: implications for birth outcomes. *Epidemiology* 4(5): 415–20.

Towner, D., Castro, M.A., Eby-Wilkens, E., Gilbert, W.M. (1999). Effect of mode of delivery in nulliparous women on neonatal intracranial injury. *New England Journal of Medicine* 341(23): 1709–14.

Townsend, C.L., Cortina-Borja, M., Peckham, C.S., de Ruiter, A., Lyall, H., Tookey, P.A. (2008). Low rates of mother-to-child transmission of HIV following effective pregnancy interventions in the United Kingdom and Ireland, 2000–2006. *AIDS* 22(8): 973–81.

Townsend, J., Wolke, D., Hayes, J. Davé, S., Rogers, C., Bloomfield, L., Quist-Therson, E., Tomlin, M., Messer, D. (2004). Routine examination of the newborn: the EMREN study. Evaluation of an extension of the midwife role including a randomised controlled trial of appropriately trained midwives and paediatric senior house officers. *Heath Technology Assessment* 8(14).

Turner Syndrome Support Society. (2009). *What is TS?* Available at http://www.tss.org.uk/what-is-ts (accessed 21 September 2009).

Tye, C., Ross, E., Kerry, M. (1988). Emergency nurse practitioner services in major accident and emergency departments: a United Kingdom postal survey. *Journal of Accident and Emergency Medicine* 15(1): 31–4.

UK National Screening Committee. (2008a). Newborn and infant physical examination. Standards and competencies. Antenatal and Newborn Screening Programmes. Available at http://newbornphysical.screening.nhs.uk/publications (accessed 11 October 2009).

UK National Screening Committee. (2008b). *NHS fetal anomaly screening programme – screening for Down's syndrome. UK NSC policy recommendations 2007–2010: model of best practice*. London, Department of Health.

US Department of Health and Human Services (USDHHS). (1990). *The health benefits of smoking cessation: a report of the Surgeon General*. DHSS Publication No. (CDC) 90–8416. Rockville, MA, Office on Smoking and Health.

Vio, F., Salazar, G., Infante, C. (1991). Smoking during pregnancy and lactation and its effects on breast milk. *American Journal of Clinical Nutrition* 54(6): 1011–16.

Wald, N.J., Cuckle, H.S., Densem, J.W., Kennard, A., Smith, D. (1992). Maternal serum screening for Down's syndrome: the effect of routine ultrasound scan determination of gestational age and adjustment for maternal weight. *British Journal of Obstetrics and Gynaecology* 99(2): 144–9.

Walker, D. (1999). Role of the routine neonatal examination (Letter). *British Medical Journal* 318(7200): 1766.

Wallace, L., Evers, K.E., Wareing, H., Dunn, O.M., Newby, K., Paiva, A., Johnson, J.L. (2007). Informing school sex education using the stages of change construct. *Journal of Health Psychology* 12(1): 179–83.

Walsh, R.A., Redman, S., Brinsmead, M.W., Byrne, J.M., Melmeth, A. (1997). A smoking cessation program at a public antenatal clinic. *American Journal of Public Health* 87(7): 1201–4.

Ward, C., Lewis, S., Coleman, T. (2007). Prevalence of maternal smoking and environmental tobacco smoke exposure during pregnancy and impact on birth weight: retrospective study using Millennium Cohort. *BMC Public Health* 7: 81.

Weitzman, M., Gortmaker, S., Klein Walker, D., Sobol, A. (1990). Maternal smoking and childhood asthma. *Pediatrics* 85(4): 505–11.

Wennerholm, U., Hagberg, H., Brorsson, B., Bergh, C. (2009). Induction of labor versus expectant management for post-date pregnancy: is there sufficient evidence for a change in clinical practice? *Acta Obstertricia et Gynecologica Scandinaviica* 88(1): 6–17.

Woollett, A. (1996). Reproductive decisions. In C. Niven, A. Walker (eds). *Conception, pregnancy and birth*. Oxford, Butterworth-Heinemann.

Wong, S., Chow, K., Ho, L. (2002). The relative risk of 'fetal distress' in pregnancy associated with meconium-stained liquor at different gestation. *Journal of Obstetrics and Gynaecology* 22(6): 294–9.

Woyton, J., Agrawal, P., Zimmer, M. (1994). Evaluation of the effect of oxytocin use for labour induction on frequency of occurrence and severity of neonatal jaundice. *Ginekologia Polska* 65(12): 682–5.

Zhang, X., Platt, R., Cnattingius, S., Joseph, K.S., Kramer, M.S. (2007). The use of customised versus population-based birth weight standards in predicting perinatal mortality. *British Journal of Obstetrics and Gynaecology* 114(4): 474–7.

Zuckerman, B., Frank, D.A., Hingson, R., Amaro, H., Levenson, S.M., Kayne, H., Parker, S., Vinci, R., Aboagye, K., Fried, L.E. (1989). Effects of maternal marijuana and cocaine use on fetal growth. *New England Journal of Medicine* 320(12): 762–8.

Zupan, J., Garner, P., Omari, A.A.A. (2004). Topical umbilical cord care at birth. *Cochrane Database of Systematic Reviews* 2: CD001057.

Index